AF598061

Security and Privacy for Implantable Medical Devices

Wayne Burleson • Sandro Carrara
Editors

Security and Privacy for Implantable Medical Devices

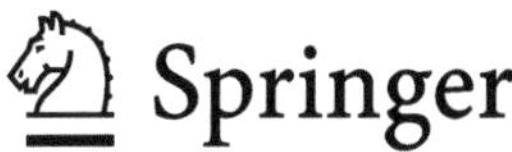

Springer

Editors
Wayne Burleson
Department of Electrical and Computer Engineering
University of Massachusetts
Amherst, MA, USA

Sandro Carrara
École Polytechnique Fédérale de Lausanne
Lausanne, Switzerland

ISBN 978-1-4614-1673-9 ISBN 978-1-4614-1674-6 (eBook)
DOI 10.1007/978-1-4614-1674-6
Springer New York Heidelberg Dordrecht London

Library of Congress Control Number: 2013948851

Printed on acid-free paper

Springer is part of Springer Science+Business Media (www.springer.com)

Contents

Chapter 1
Introduction

Wayne Burleson and Sandro Carrara

Implantable medical devices (IMDs) have advanced considerably in the last few decades, promising unprecedented access to the human body to gather personal health data anywhere and any time. Widely deployed devices such as pacemakers and insulin pumps already provide enormous health benefits. Cochlear and ocular implants use advanced microelectronics and novel powering schemes for vastly improved hearing and vision. Biosensors address disease by drug and biomarker detection with myriad applications, ranging from cancer therapies and infectious disease detection to genome analysis, promising to improve health, increase safety, and reduce the cost of diagnostics.

However, the security and privacy of these devices and their data have still not been adequately addressed. The low cost and lightweight nature of the devices makes implementation of standard information security and cryptography challenging and motivates novel approaches that are customized to constraints and threat models. Wireless interfaces are perhaps the most obvious vulnerability; however, device counterfeiting and data fraud are also realistic threats. The most disturbing concerns arise in systems where drug (e.g., insulin pumps) or electric therapies (e.g., pacemakers) can be maliciously modified to deliver lethal results. But the security and privacy of personal health data and genomics information motivate discussions about data ownership and fundamental human privacy rights.

Most recently, the development of new biosensors has allowed blood tests to be performed in the body that previously required blood sampling, incurring costs, compromising safety, and causing inconvenience for patient and physician. Furthermore, the fact that lab tests can be performed anywhere and any time allows

W. Burleson (✉)
Department of Electrical and Computer Engineering, University of Massachusetts,
309C Knowles Engineering Building, Amherst 01003, USA
e-mail: Burleson@ecs.umass.edu

S. Carrara
École Polytechnique Fédérale de Lausanne, Lausanne, Switzerland
e-mail: Sandro.Carrara@epfl.ch

W. Burleson and S. Carrara (eds.), *Security and Privacy for Implantable Medical Devices*,
DOI 10.1007/978-1-4614-1674-6_1,

unprecedented exposure of the body and personal health information. Personalized health solutions can be used to tackle difficult problems in cancer and other therapies. Responses to drugs and drug interactions can be monitored on a much finer-grained level than before.

However, the increased reliance on these technologies, especially in the case of potentially life-saving therapies, can introduce difficult tradeoffs in reliability and security. Personal health information that was once restricted to the confines of a medical laboratory and physician could now potentially be accessible to various unauthorized parties.

Wireless Access to Implantable Devices: A Double-Edged Sword

Wireless connectivity at various scales provides numerous benefits with respect to implantable medical devices (IMDs). The ability to communicate with an implanted device allows data to be transferred both up and down as well as download of control information and software updates. Fortunately, most data transfer rates from IMDs are quite slow and the out-of-body radio can be located quite close, removing many concerns about power levels and eavesdropping. Recent examples where the external radio is on a bandage [1] just millimeters from a subcutaneous implant [2] pose issues that are relatively easy to solve in terms of wireless communication system design by drawing upon recent techniques in radio-frequency identification (RFID), (NFC), and inductive coupling. More challenging are deeply implanted devices that must cross significant amounts of human tissue before leaving the body. Examples include deep brain implants, deep heart implants, and fetal monitors [3].

If the external radio is on the body (Fig. 1.1), this can either tie into or form the basis of a body area network (BAN). BANs have been proposed for a wide range of applications, and a good survey on them can be found in [4]. The IEEE recently announced a new standard for BANs (the IEEE 802.15.6) that emphasizes ultra-low-power devices.

Wireless connectivity also provides capabilities for directly updating electronic health records (EHRs) [5]. One of the main concerns about EHRs has been the cost and accuracy of manual data entry [6]. By directly entering data from implantable devices, some of these concerns may be reduced. In addition, wireless capabilities facilitate the concept of a personal health record (PHR) or portfolio (PHP) [7], which extends the EHR to a record that is under the control of the patient. This addresses many concerns about individual civil liberties and privacy rights.

If the external radio is not on the body, the wireless communication problem is significantly more challenging and additional vulnerabilities arise. However, this scenario is quite attractive because it avoids the inconvenience of the patients having to wear a device, possibly losing the device, and keeping it powered. Instead, a wall-powered base station, similar to a Wi-Fi router, can be used to communicate

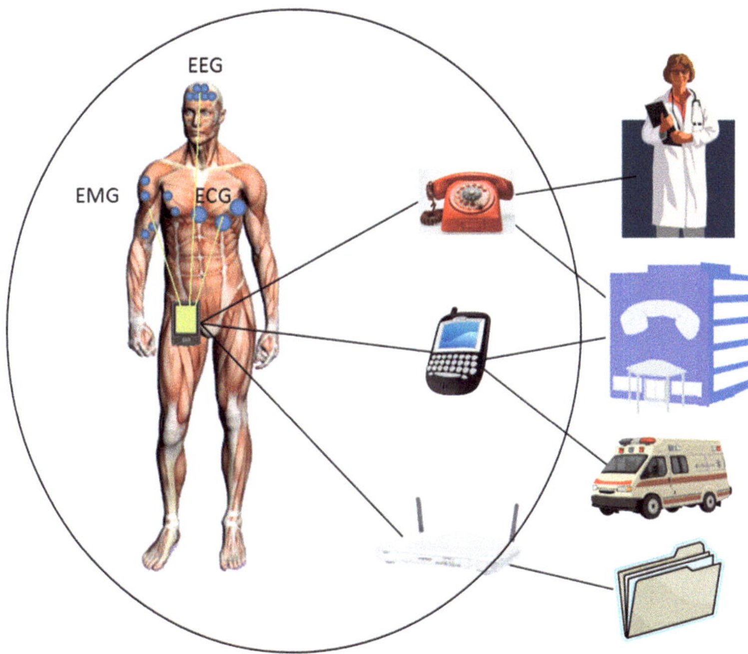

Fig. 1.1 A body area network (BAN) connects various sensors to a wearable router/hub that communicates wirelessly with other networks for medical, emergency, and record-keeping purposes (Courtesy of CSEM/Switzerland)

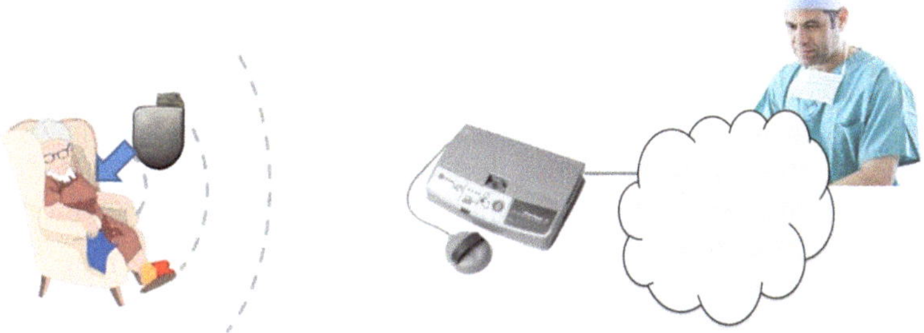

Fig. 1.2 Remote access to implantable pacemaker and cardiac monitor (Courtesy of Golkatta (MIT))

with the implanted device and then directly tie into the cellular or fixed network and then to the Internet (Fig. 1.2). A recent US study suggests that physician access to medical devices through remote monitoring can offer a reduction in hospital visits by 40 % and cost per visit by US$1,800 [8].

Wireless powering is another advantage of wireless access to subcutaneous IMDs (Fig. 1.3). Although numerous possibilities have been proposed for energy

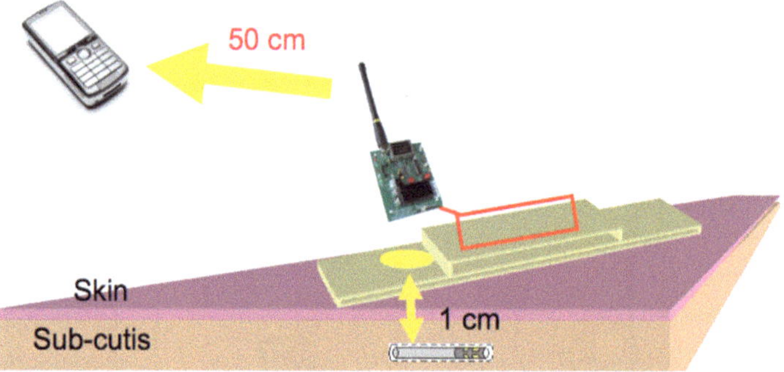

Fig. 1.3 Fully implantable medical devices may be powered by patches located on top of the skin, and these electronic patches may be wirelessly connected to a smartphone via a Bluetooth link

harvesting within the body, including thermal gradients, electrochemical techniques, and vibration harvesting, most are not considered sufficiently mature or reliable for medical applications [9]. Batteries have their own problems, including size, weight, cost, and toxicity. Most rechargeable batteries have safety risks, which limit their application in implantable devices. Recent problems with lithium-ion batteries in various applications will only continue to hinder their public acceptance for safety-critical applications like medical devices. A major reason for pacemaker replacement surgery is simply due to the lifetime of the battery (approximately 7–10 years), so any reduction in power consumption can translate to reduced surgery. Wireless powering over a short range, similar to RFID and smart-card technology, is very promising for providing up to milliwatts of power to the implantable device. Recent research [10] has shown that optimal powering frequencies in GHz range allow very small millimeter-sized antennas on implantable devices. We have demonstrated novel antennas for remote powering from patches applied to the skin directly above a subcutaneous device that allow MHz frequencies, too, for millimeter-sized antennas on implantable devices [1]. The close proximity and ease of alignment allow highly efficient energy transfer.

The Promise of Implantable Medical Devices

This book will show that IMDs are not limited to biosensors. Chapter 5 shows a quite different case of IMDs, and numerous other IMDs are on the drawing boards. Therefore, a taxonomy of IMDs can be defined by several dimensions:

- Physical location/depth, procedure, lifetime;
- Sensing/actuating functions (sense, deliver drugs or stimulus, grow tissue!);
- Computational capabilities;
- Data storage (both volatile and non-volatile);

- Communication: bandwidth, up-link, down-link, interdevice positioning system (IPS), distance to reader, noise;
- Energy requirements (memory, communication, computation), powering, harvesting, storage (battery or capacitive);
- Vulnerabilities: security functions (access control, authentication, encryption);
- Reliability and failure modes.

Of course, IMDs may be formalized in the abstract, as a general concept. However, the aim of this book is more to provide an introduction to the field of IMDs and to related fields in security and privacy. Therefore, we will introduce here the notion of the promise of biosensors by considering some key examples the details of which will be presented and discussed in more depth in Chaps. 2, 3, and 5. Thus, here we briefly touch on a few example devices, from those already on the market to those from the literature at the cutting edge and state of the art in medical implants.

Modern medicine is currently facing new challenges. One in particular is of importance for this book: *the personalization of pharmacological therapies offered to patients*. This new challenge is now trying to address the main problem in pharmacological therapy: when a group of patients is treated with exactly the same pharmacological compound, the result is usually different in terms of patient responses (for more details, see the introduction in Chap. 4). The market already tried once to solve this problem with a new chip based on microarray technology and capable of clustering patients into different groups [11]. The aim was to cluster patients in order to forecast their behaviors in terms of their response to the same therapy. However, this approach has been not very successful. The reason is not related to the chip performance but to the nature of genetics. Patients are different not only at the level of gene expression. They are also different from each other at the level of gene regulation, epigenetics, and daily variations in their metabolism. Therefore, daily monitoring of their metabolism is strictly required if the new approach of therapy personalization hopes to succeed.

In fact, that approach is already in place for diabetic patients. As amply shown in Chap. 2, glucose control is the cornerstone of diabetes mellitus (DM) treatment. Continuous glucose monitoring systems provide a dynamic assessment of shifting blood glucose concentrations and facilitate the making of optimal treatment decisions for diabetic patients. These systems contribute to the management of glycemic control and personalize insulin administration. Such an approach permits the narrowing of daily glucose fluctuations in blood while decreasing the incidence of hypoglycemic phenomena. This aspect is of key importance because improved glycemic control has proven beneficial to patients – and to the healthcare economy – by reducing the frequency and severity of associated complications. Glycemic control is now also gaining importance in intensive care units. It significantly improves both mortality and morbidity but requires frequent (often hourly) and accurate glucose testing. Therefore, a new generation of intravenous glucose systems are presently under development in key biosensor companies [12], such as A. Menarini Diagnostics, whose technologists contributed Chap. 2 of this book.

Another improvement in the human telemetry of glucose monitoring is the possibility of having remote access to data gathered by the measurement system. As shown in Chap. 3, wireless potentiostats are now being developed and commercialized for use in the development of implantable electrochemical biosensors for the monitoring of physiological markers in a wide range of pathologies. Chapter 3 presents an example of those developments by discussing the merits and drawbacks of a novel implantable biotransducer, the dual responsive MDEA 5037 of ABTECH Scientific [13]. The chapter refers to a series of laboratory tests that have shown positive assays on the device performance. For implantable amperometric biosensors, this system fulfills the desired functionality in the most efficient way possible, also giving due consideration to size, power management, telemetry capabilities, and signal processing. Therefore, it holds good promise for future devices in the market for metabolite telemetry.

Of course, in attempting to develop a monitoring system that can follow human metabolism over time, we are confronted with two main issues: providing the right specificity and the right sensitivity. Chapter 4 of this book provides a general overview on the possibility of developing devices that not only assure glycemia monitoring but also monitoring of glucose, lactate, adenosine triphosphate (ATP), bilirubin, and many other substances that are strictly related to several well-known human diseases. The chapter also presents a series of technological approaches that have been used in recent years in the successful development of a fully implantable subcutaneous implant that assures the metabolism monitoring of humans and addresses issues concerning the biocompatibility of those kinds of implants [15].

Problem of Specificity

When planning the development of an implantable device capable of detecting several molecules related to human metabolism, it is necessary to be able to identify the proper probes that can provide specific recognition of each single target metabolite. Chapter 4 of this book deals with specific recognition and discusses several possibilities: antibodies, oxidases, hexokinases, and cytochromes. Antibodies are the first molecules to consider when referring to specific molecular recognition. However, they are not very suitable for continuous monitoring for the following reason. When a sensing surface is fabricated based on an antibody, the obtained sensor is an immune sensor capable of sensing antigens (the target molecules of an antibody); meanwhile they are trapped by the antibodies that had previously been immobilized on the surface. Of course, the senseing is "continuous" but it applies only until the surface is fully saturated. Once all the antibodies have stuck to the antigen, they are no longer able to monitor other antigens arriving at the sensing surface. Thus, the surface is the sensing is continuous. Instead, enzymes are proteins too with the capability of true continuous monitoring because they are biological catalysts that are free to work on other substrates (the target molecules of an enzyme) immediately after participating in the previous reaction. Thus, enzymes are always prepared to deal with new incoming substrates at the sensing surface. Hence, the surface is constantly ready to detect new target molecules. Chapter 4 introduces three types of possible enzymes for continuous monitoring: oxidases, which are usually used to detect glucose (the glycemic blood level), lactate, cholesterol, and many other endogenous metabolites; hexokinases, usually used to detect endogenous molecules that do not have a corresponding oxidase (the chapter presents the case of the ATP); and cytochromes, which have been proposed for the detection of several commonly used drug compounds and which were recently successfully introduced for continuous monitoring in personalized therapy [15].

Problem of Sensitivity

Generic amperometric sensors respond to increases in the amount of molecular concentration by an increase in currents. However, all sensors typically become blind below a certain concentration. The minimum amount of molecules that return the first slightest increase of current in a sensor is usually called the *detection limit*. Of course, the detection limit is a crucial parameter for identifying the working technology considering our goals. In fact, if the detection limit of a sensor does not fit within the physiological or pharmacological ranges of the molecules we would like to detect, we completely lose the possibility of addressing the medical application of our sensor. Chapter 4 also presents and discusses in detail how to use nanomaterials to improve the sensitivity of electrochemical sensors and, thus, how to decrease their detection limits in order to optimally use these kinds of sensors in the most important biomedical applications of IMDs. The nanotechnology proposed in Chap. 4 consists mainly of carbon nanotubes that have been successfully employed to enhance the sensor properties of both endogenous (e.g., glucose [16]) and exogenous metabolites (e.g., anticancer and anti-inflammatory drugs [17]).

Another Kind of Medical Implant

Part I of this book, "The Promise of IMDs," closes with a completely different kind of IMD: Chap. 5 refers to the possibility of developing IMDs that provide in vivo bioreactors. This kind of IMD addresses the human aspiration of creating our own tissue and organ substitutes. The last approach proposed for that purpose involved harvesting cells from the human organism (so-called stem cells) and expanding them in vitro before seeding them onto a biodegradable scaffold shaped according to the contour of the tissue to be replaced. The cell-scaffold construct is usually cultured in an in vitro bioreactor that tries to mimic the in vivo regenerative niche. Although successful in some cases (the typical successful example is that of corneal cells), the approach has several disadvantages and technical obstacles inherent in the conventional tissue-engineering process. Therefore, a new approach has emerged involving the design of in vivo bioreactors. These completely new kinds of IMD are mainly implanted engineered tissues supported by an intrascaffold flow of medium created by an extracorporeal portable pump system for in situ tissue and organ regeneration. This design combines the traditionally separated in vitro three-dimensional cell-scaffold culture system and the in vivo regenerative processes associated with engineered tissue while treating recipients as bioreactors for tissue-engineered prostheses. Of course, it is very easy to imagine that marketing such an innovative technology would require automated systems also capable of hosting all the required fluidics [18] and carriers [19], as well as new monitoring sensors, in order to precisely control the tissue regeneration.

Security in Implantable Medical Devices

The second part of this book provides an introduction to security issues related to IMDs. Security is defined as the protection of a device, system, or data from a malicious (and usually human) adversary [20]. This should be distinguished from safety, where problems arise due to design errors, system failures, or random acts. However, IMD security is more complex than information security because it involves a physical system and humans as both producers and consumers of data. The relatively new discipline of security engineering [21] has much to offer in addressing this issue and provides a systematic approach. The methods of security engineering involve identifying the following aspects:

- Assets
- Vulnerabilities
- Threats
- Defenses

Defenses can be further divided into:

- Policies
- Mechanisms
- Enforcement

Security engineering is a challenging problem that is compounded by a variety of myths that include the following:

- Security is binary
- Standards are infallible
- Penetration testing and security consultants can ensure security

These problems arise primarily due to the fact that the adversary is human and attacks continue to evolve and improve to avoid new defenses. An escalating game of cat and mouse ensues. The adversary has the advantage by only needing to find a single point of weakness, while the defender must ensure that all possible attacks are defended. The multilayered nature of embedded computing systems further exacerbates the problem, and it is in fact between layers where many attacks succeed. This is due to the limitations of models and abstractions that were often designed without security in mind. Hardware-based attacks are an example, where information leaks through power and timing side channels not envisioned at the time of design [22].

Security guru and blogger Bruce Schneier [23] reminds us that:

> Any person can invent a security system so clever that he or she can't imagine a way of breaking it.

Schneier criticizes security approaches that only try to prevent intrusion, instead arguing that it is more important to design systems to fail well. This has become a standard approach in large-scale cybersecurity, including military and financial systems, where a certain amount of intrusion is assumed and the objectives are containment and resiliency. These arguments can be extended to medical systems, where the ultimate assets are human life and safety.

Respected security and cryptography expert Ari Juels [24] proposes the following tenets:

- Security should be designed in rather than added on. The example of the Internet illustrates this rather painfully.
- Open design: Public scrutiny usually breeds stronger systems than private finger crossing. Openness has long been a cardinal rule of cryptography and a pillar of secure system design. Similarly, responsible disclosure of vulnerabilities holds the technology industry to high standards and brings vital education to the community.
- Security should be designed holistically because piecewise solutions inevitably leave gaps at their boundaries.

These points will be expanded in Chaps. 7 and 8, which were written by leading security experts. Chapter 7 emphasizes the challenges associated with securing IMDs. The chapter presents some standard recommendations for sound security design and applies them to three classes of IMDs. Chapter 8 focuses on the wireless aspect of IMDs and their interface with BANs. Several attacks are shown and countermeasures proposed. Although by no means exhaustive, the novel attacks illustrate in detail the complexity and ingenuity that characterize modern threat scenarios. The reader is encouraged to expand on these two chapters by envisioning more sophisticated threats and the wide range of issues that must be considered in security engineering.

References

1. Jacopo Olivo, Sandro Carrara, and Giovanni De Micheli, *A study of Multi-Layer Spiral Inductors for Remote Powering of Implantable Sensors*, IEEE Transaction of Biomedical Circuits and Systems, 2013, in press
2. Sandro Carrara, Andrea Cavallini, Sara Ghoreishizadeh, Jacopo Olivo, Giovanni De Micheli, Developing Highly-Integrated Subcutaneous Biochips for Remote Monitoring of Human Metabolism, IEEE Sensors conference 2012, Taipei, Taiwan, October 28–31, 2012, p. 271–274
3. Benjamin Cotté, Cyril Lafon, Catherine Dehollain, and Jean-yves Chapelon. Theoretical Study for Safe and Efficient Energy Transfer to Deeply Implanted Devices Using Ultrasound. IEEE Transactions on Ultrasonics, Ferroelectrics, and Frequency Control, vol. 59, no. 8, August 2012
4. Gyselinckx, B., Van Hoof, C.; Ryckaert, J.; Yazicioglu, R.F.; Fiorini, P.; Leonov, V., "Human++: Autonomous Wireless Sensors for Body Area Networks," IEEE 2005 Custom Integrated Circuits Conference, pp. 13–19
5. Bruce Moulton, Zenon Chaczko, Mark Karatovic, Updating Electronic Health Records with Information from Sensor Systems: Considerations Relating To Standards and Architecture Arising From the Development of a Prototype System, Journal of Convergence Information Technology Volume 4, Number 4, December 2009, pp. 21–26
6. S. Kliff, Why electronic health records failed? washingtonpost.com, Jan 11, 2013
7. http://personalhealthportfolio.wordpress.com/
8. Wayne Burleson, Design Challenges for Secure Implantable Medical Devices, seminar published at http://www.cs.ru.nl/ifip-wg11.2/events/Slides-seminar2012/Burleson.pdf
9. Jacopo Olivo, Sandro Carrara, Giovanni De Micheli, *Energy Harvesting and Remote Powering for Implantable Biosensors*, IEEE Sensors Journal, 11(2011), 1573–1586
10. A. Poon, S. O'Driscoll, and T.Meng, "Optimal Operating Frequency in Wireless Power Transmission for Implantable Devices," Proceedings of the 29th Annual International Conference of the IEEE EMBS, pp.5673–5678, 2007
11. De Leon, J., Susce, M., Murray-Carmichael, E., The AmpliChip CYP450 genotyping test: Integrating a new clinical tool,Mol. Diagn. Ther. 10 (2006), 135–151
12. Valgimigli, F. Lucarelli, C. Scuffi, S. Morandi, and I. Sposato, "Eval- uating the clinical accuracy of GlucoMenDay: A novel microdialysis- based continuous glucose monitor," *J. Diabetes Sci. Technol.,* vol. 4, no. 5, pp. 1182–1192, 2010
13. Rahman, A.R.A., G. Justin, and A. Guiseppi-Elie, *Towards an implantable biochip for glucose and lactate monitoring using microdisc electrode arrays (MDEAs).* Biomedical Microdevices, 2009. **11**(1): p. 75–85
14. Sandro Carrara, Sara Seyedeh Ghoreishizadeh, Jacopo Olivo, Irene Taurino, Camilla Baj-Rossi, Andrea Cavallini, Maaike Op de Beeck, Catherine Dehollain, Wayne Burleson, Francis Gabriel Moussy, Anthony Guiseppi-Elie, Giovanni De Micheli, *Fully Integrated Biochip Platforms for Advanced Healthcare*, Sensors 12(2012) 11013–11060
15. Camilla Baj-Rossi, Giovanni De Micheli, Sandro Carrara, Continuous monitoring of a drug in real-time by a cytochrome P450-based electrochemical sensor, Biosensors and Bioelectronics, 2013, submitted
16. Guiseppi-Elie, A.; Lei, C.; Baughman, R.H. Direct electron transfer to glucose oxidase using carbon nanotubes. *Nanotechnology* **2002**, *13,* 559–564
17. Sandro Carrara, Andrea Cavallini, Victor Erokhin, Giovanni De Micheli, *Multi-panel drugs detection in human serum for personalized therapy*, Biosensors and Bioelectronics, 26 (2011) 3914–3919
18. Tan Q, Hillinger S,van Blitterswijk CA, Weer W. Intra-scaffold continuous medium flow combines chondrocyte seeding and culture systems for tissue engineered trachea construction. Interact Cardiovasc Thorac Surg. 2009 Jan;8(1):27–30

19. Tan Q, El-Badry A, Contaldo C, Steiner R, Hillinger S, Welti M, Spahn D, Higuera G, van Blitterswjik C, Luo QQ, Weder W. The effect of perfluorocarbon-based artificial oxygen carriers on tissue-engineered trachea. Tissue Eng. 2009 Sep;15(9):2471–80
20. Matt Bishop, Computer Security: Art and Science, Addison-Wesley Publisher, December 2002
21. R. Anderson, Security Engineering, Wiley, 2010, available free on-line (http://www.cl.cam.ac.uk/~rja14/book.html)
22. C. Kocher, Timing Attacks on Implementations of Diffie-Hellman, RSA, DSS, and Other Systems, Online, (available free on-line http://www.cryptography.com/resources/ whitepapers/TimingAttacks.pdf)
23. http://www.schneier.com/
24. Ari Juels, personal communication, 2008.

Part I

Chapter 2
Blood Glucose Monitoring Systems

Francesco Valgimigli, Fabrizio Mastrantonio, and Fausto Lucarelli

Background and Content of This Chapter

Glucose control is the cornerstone of diabetes mellitus (DM) treatment. Although self-monitoring of blood glucose (SMBG) still remains the best procedure in clinical practise, continuous glucose monitoring systems (CGMSs) provide a dynamic assessment of shifting blood glucose concentrations and facilitate the making of optimal treatment decisions for the diabetic patient. As such, CGM systems could contribute to a paradigm shift in the management of glycaemic control, making insulin administration more personalised. Such an approach makes it possible to narrow the daily glucose fluctuations in blood whilst decreasing the incidence of hypoglycaemic phenomena. This aspect is of paramount importance because improved glycaemic control has been shown to be beneficial to patients – and to the healthcare industry– by reducing the frequency and severity of associated complications [55]. Moreover, tight glycaemic control (TGC) in acutely ill hospitalised patients significantly improves both mortality and morbidity but requires frequent (often hourly) and accurate glucose testing [32, 33]. To meet the specific needs of intensive care units ICUs, specifically designed glucose hospital meters are already commercially available whilst a new generation of intravascular CGM systems is presently under development and clinical testing.

The aim of this document is to review the principles underlying the use of electrochemical glucose biosensors for monitoring the blood glucose level in diabetic patients.

The introductory section provides descriptions of blood, general features of the enzymatic systems and basic carbohydrate chemistry. The concept of the biosensor is introduced while focusing on the enzymes that represent the heart of essentially all commercially available glucosensors: glucose oxidase (GOD) and glucose dehydrogenases (GDHs).

F. Valgimigli (✉) • F. Mastrantonio • F. Lucarelli
A. Menarini Diagnostics, Florence, Italy
e-mail: fvalgimigli@menarini.it; fmastrantonio@menarini.it; flucarelli@menarini.it

W. Burleson and S. Carrara (eds.), *Security and Privacy for Implantable Medical Devices*, DOI 10.1007/978-1-4614-1674-6_2,

The working principles of the so-called mediator-less and mediator-based electrochemical glucosensors are then described. Special emphasis is given to those factors – both physical (environmental) and (bio) chemical – that affect the accuracy and precision of blood glucose quantisation.

The mechanism by which the most common endogenous or exogenous compounds interfere is discussed in relation to which element of the glucosensor architecture (i.e. electrode, mediator or enzyme) is directly involved.

The final sections discuss continuous glucose monitoring in terms of its purposes, technologies, target population, accuracy, clinical-indication outcomes and problems. In this context, the most promising advancements in CGMSs, such as methods for non-invasive continuous monitoring and fully implantable biosensors, are reported. The commercial advent of the aforementioned technologies will enable diabetic patients to use CGMSs more routinely than ever before.

Introduction

Diabetes mellitus is a worldwide public threat and is expected to become one of the major healthcare challenges in the new millennium. Recently compiled data by the World Health Organization (WHO) shows that worldwide approximately 180 million people have diabetes and that this number may double by the year 2025. This metabolic disorder results from an insulin lack (T1DM) or deficiency (T2DM) that causes blood glucose concentrations to reach levels that are higher than the normal range of 80–120 mg/dL (4.4–6.6 mM) [1]. More specifically, in Type 1 diabetes (T1DM) the pancreas fails to produce insulin, which is essential for survival. This form of diabetes develops most frequently in children and adolescents but is being increasingly diagnosed later in life. In contrast, Type 2 diabetes (T2DM) results from the body's inability to respond properly to the action of insulin produced by the pancreas. T2DM is much more common than T1DM and accounts for around 90% of all diabetes cases worldwide. It occurs most frequently in adults but is being noted increasingly in adolescents as well. Certain genetic markers have been shown to increase the risk of developing T1DM. T2DM is strongly familiar, but it is only recently that some genes have been consistently associated with increased risk for developing Type 2 diabetes in certain populations. Both types of diabetes are complex diseases caused by mutations in more than one gene as well as by environmental factors. It is worth pointing out that the last 20 years have seen an explosive increase in diabetes globally linked to, among other factors, the emergence of obesity (diabesity). Diabetes has been recognised as the fourth leading cause of death and disability in the world. The disease is always associated, in the medium to long term, with the occurrence of multi-organ complications such as diabetic retinopathy, nephropathy, and neuropathy, mostly related to lifestyle, treatment and poor glycaemic metabolism control. The American Diabetes Association (ADA) Guidelines recommend a close monitoring of the blood glucose in order to prevent,

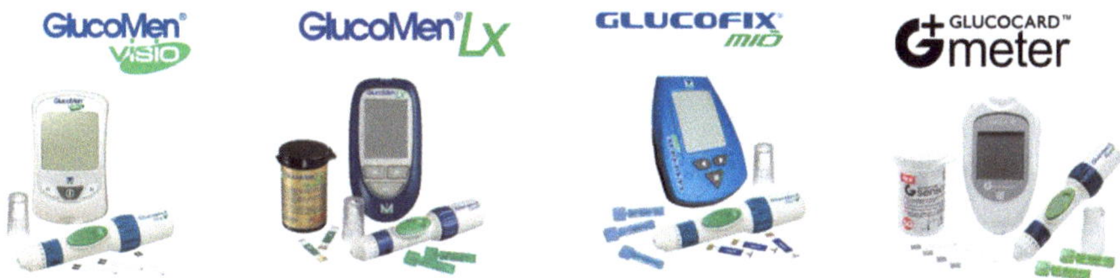

Fig. 2.1 Examples of glucometers for diabetes self-testing

reduce or delay the onset of such complications. Accordingly, millions of diabetics test their blood glucose levels daily, making glucose the most commonly measured analyte. The most important support to this practice is represented by commercial *glucometers* (e.g. Fig. 2.1), low-cost yet highly specific and sensitive analytical devices.

The tremendous economic burden associated with the management of diabetes, along with the challenge of providing such reliable and tight glycaemic control, has thus led to a considerable amount of research and innovative detection strategies [1, 2].

Definitions

Whole Blood, Blood Serum and Blood Plasma

Blood is the specialised bodily fluid that delivers all necessary substances (i.e. nutrients and oxygen) to the body's cells and transports the waste products away. Whole blood is composed of *blood cells* suspended in a liquid called *blood plasma* (Fig. 2.2).

Blood Cells

The blood cells present in blood are mainly red blood cells (also called RBCs or erythrocytes), white blood cells (leukocytes) and thrombocytes. One microlitre of blood typically contains the following substances:

(I) 4.7–6.1 million (male) or 4.2–5.4 million (female) erythrocytes. The RBCs contain haemoglobin, an iron-containing protein that reversibly binds oxygen, facilitating its transport throughout the body. RBCs are also marked by glycoproteins, which define the different blood types. The proportion of blood occupied by RBCs is referred to as the haematocrit, and is normally approximately 45%.

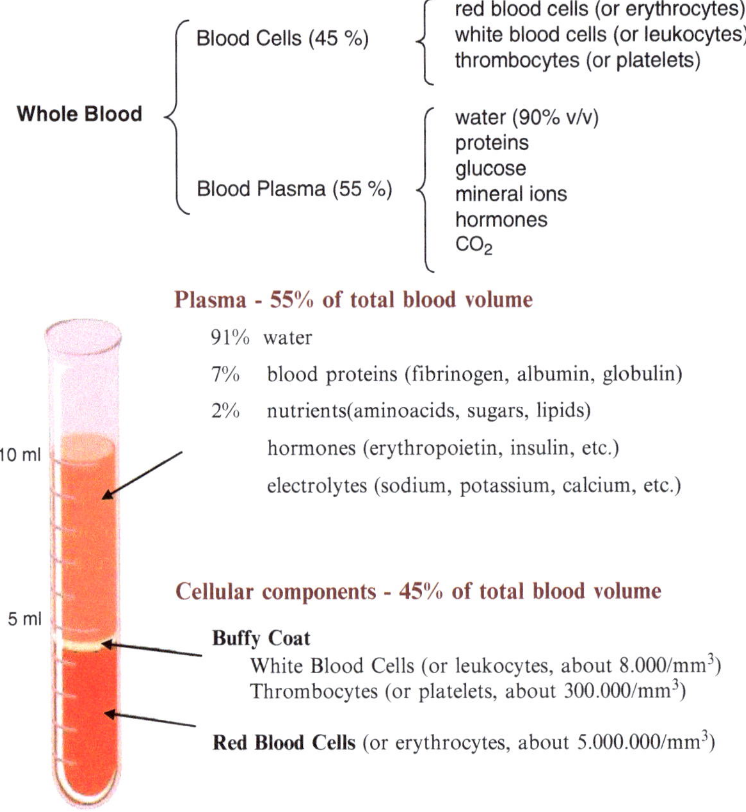

Fig. 2.2 Composition of a typical blood sample

(II) 4,000–11,000 leukocytes. White blood cells are part of the immune system; they destroy and remove old or aberrant cells and attack infectious agents (pathogens) and foreign substances.

(III) 200,000–500,000 thrombocytes. Thrombocytes, also called platelets, are responsible for blood clotting (coagulation). They change fibrinogen into fibrin. This fibrin creates a mesh onto which RBCs collect and clot, which then stops more blood from leaving the body and also helps to prevent bacteria from entering in.

Blood Plasma

Approximately 55% of total blood volume is blood plasma, a fluid that is itself straw-yellow in colour. Blood plasma is essentially an aqueous solution containing 90% water, 8% proteins and trace amounts of other materials. Plasma circulates

Table 2.1 Physico-chemical characteristics of a normal arterial blood sample

Parameter	Value
Haematocrit	(38 ÷ 52)% for males (37 ÷ 47)% for females
pH	7.35 ÷ 7.45
PO_2	10 ÷ 13 kPa (80 ÷ 100 mmHg)
PCO_2	4.8 ÷ 5.8 kPa (35 ÷ 45 mmHg)
HCO_3^-	21 mM ÷ 27 mM
Oxygen saturation	Oxygenated: 98 ÷ 99% Deoxygenated: 75%

Table 2.2 Typical oxygenation of various blood types

Blood sample	Mean pO_2 mmHg	pO_2 range mmHg
Arterial	95	75–120
Capillary	75	60–90
Venous	50	30–70
Venous aged	15–20	5–30
O_2 therapy	variable	>100–600

dissolved nutrients, such as glucose, amino acids and fatty acids (either dissolved into the blood or bound to plasma proteins), and removes waste products, such as carbon dioxide, urea and lactic acid.

Other important components of plasma include:

- Serum albumin
- Blood-clotting factors (to facilitate coagulation)
- Immunoglobulins (antibodies)
- Lipoprotein particles
- Other proteins
- Electrolytes (mainly sodium and chloride ions)

Blood plasma is prepared by spinning a tube of fresh whole blood in a centrifuge until the blood cells fall to the bottom of the tube.

Blood Serum

The term serum refers to plasma from which the clotting proteins have been removed. Most of the proteins remaining are albumin and immunoglobulins.

Physico-chemical Characteristics of Different Blood Types

Several important physico-chemical characteristics of different types of blood are listed in Tables 2.1 and 2.2.

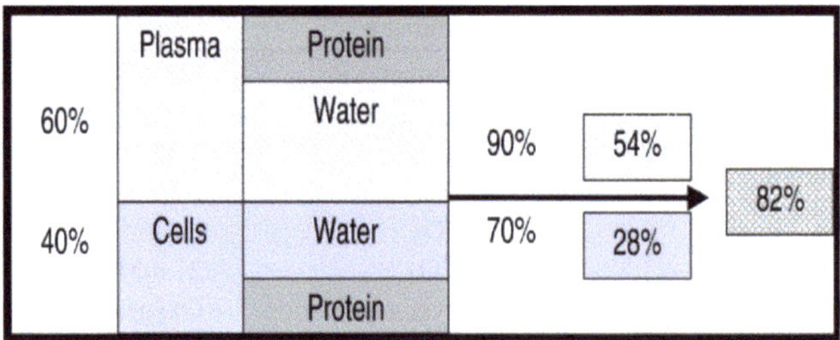

Fig. 2.3 Relative water content of whole blood and blood plasma

Blood Glucose

Blood glucose levels can be quantified using both small handheld analysers and bulky laboratory instruments. All glucometers are calibrated against plasma but can quantify glucose exclusively using whole blood samples. In contrast, in clinical chemistry labs glucose can be measured on serum, plasma and whole blood.

Blood plasma is prepared by spinning a tube of fresh whole blood in a centrifuge until the blood cells fall to the bottom of the tube. This procedure avoids the consumption of glucose by red cells, which would lead to an underestimation of blood glucose values compared to the 'fresh' sample. When whole blood is the preferred sample, its coagulation must be prevented by adding anticoagulants such as etilendiamminotetraacetic acid (EDTA), heparin, or oxalate. It is also recommended to add fluorides as glycolysis inhibitors because cell glycolysis would deplete the glucose concentration by approximately 5%/h.

Capillary blood glucose concentrations are higher than venous blood glucose ones because the glucose in capillary blood has not been fully delivered to the cells yet. Venous blood glucose levels are approximately 10% lower than arterial blood glucose levels.

The concentration of glucose in whole blood is approximately 10–15% lower than the concentration of glucose measured in plasma or serum. This can be understood in terms of steric considerations and according to the following example (Fig. 2.3).

In this example, the haematocrit is 40% and the water content for the fraction 'cells' is approximately 70%. The total water content of this fraction is, therefore, 28% of the total whole blood volume. From the 60% plasma volume, 90% is water, thus giving a water content of 54% for the plasma portion of the whole blood. Thus, the total water content of whole blood is 82% (54% + 28%). In these conditions, the plasma/whole blood ratio of water content is $0.9/0.82 = 1.10$, which reflects the 10% higher glucose values in plasma compared to whole blood [3, 4].

Biosensors

A biosensor is an analytical device in which a biological recognition element is combined with a physico-chemical transducer. It normally consists of three parts:

(I) The *biological sensing element* (capable of specifically interacting with the target molecule);
(II) The *transducer* (i.e. the element that converts the biorecognition event into a measurable signal);
(III) The *associated electronics* or signal processor (i.e. the element that is primarily responsible for displaying the results in a user-friendly way).

Biosensing element. Typically, the biological sensing elements employed by glucose biosensors are the same enzymes that cells use for the normal metabolism of this carbohydrate: GOD and GDH. The use of either engineered enzymes and synthetic receptors (e.g. boronic acid functionalised surfaces) has also been reported. However, discussion of the advantages and disadvantages of glucose-specific synthetic receptors goes beyond the purpose of this report.

Transducer. As the field of biosensors has been the subject of intense investigations in recent decades, essentially all possible physico-chemical transducers have already been explored for the conversion of a given biorecognition event into a measurable signal. Such transducers include electrochemical, optical and gravimetric sensors. Nowadays, however, the majority of home blood glucose meters relies on electrochemical measuring principles (Fig. 2.4).

In these cases, the biosensor is an electrochemical cell formed by at least a reference electrode and an enzyme (either GOD or GDH)-functionalised working electrode. The presence of glucose into the sample stimulates the enzyme activity with the consequent generation of an electrochemically active compound (e.g. H_2O_2). Detection of this compound (whose concentration is directly proportional to the original concentration of glucose) is, then, typically carried out by amperometry. This electrochemical technique relies on the application of a properly chosen (and constant) difference of potential between the reference and the working electrode. The current that results from the reaction induced by the applied potential represents the analytical signal.

In the plethora of available methods, any given strategy has its own points of strength and weakness, associated with specific elements of the biosensing path. According to Fig. 2.4, these elements include an enzyme/coenzyme pair, electrochemical mediator (where used) and electrode transducer. The precision and accuracy of glucose determinations are also a direct function of the ability of the sensor to suppress any possible interference. The interferents can act at different levels of the biosensor architecture. For example, the enzyme can exhibit non-specific interaction with sugars other than glucose. The oxygen itself, an essential enzyme cosubstrate for non-mediated systems, can be seen as an interferent when artificial electron acceptors (i.e. mediators such as potassium ferricyanide) are employed. A number of endogenous or exogenous compounds can also interfere with the

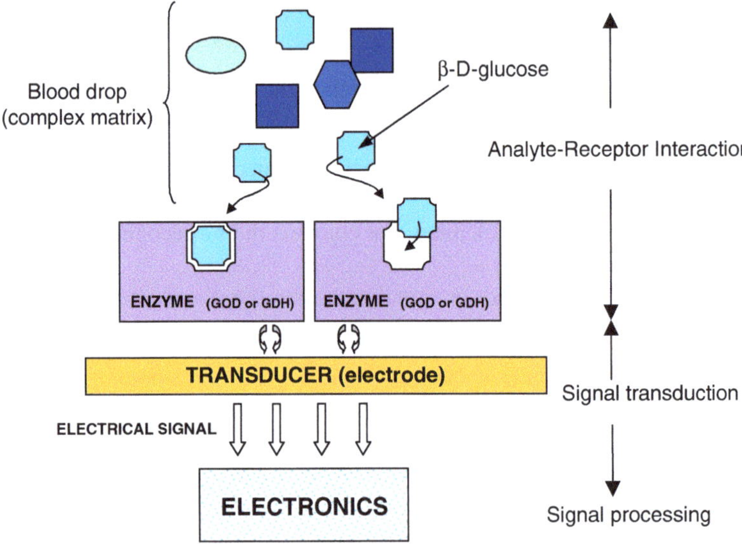

Fig. 2.4 Scheme of an electrochemical glucose biosensor. The glucose oxidase (GOD) (or glucose dehydrogenase [GDH]) enzyme (biological recognition element or receptor) is able to specifically recognise the analyte (β-D-glucose) even when the latter must be found in a blood sample (i.e. a highly complex matrix). This biorecognition event results in the generation of an electrical current, which is measured by the meter, and then further converted into the glucose concentration result

electrochemical detection step. This is, for example, the case with compounds such as ascorbic acid (which can directly exchange electrons at the electrode surface) or haematocrit (which, because of its corpuscular nature, interferes by modifying, for example, the available active area of the sensor or the fluidity of the sample).

Enzymes

General Features

Enzymes are biomolecules that catalyse (i.e. increase the rate of) chemical reactions [5]. Enzymes are globular proteins whose activity is determined by their three-dimensional structure (Fig. 2.5).

Each unique amino acid sequence produces a specific structure with unique properties. Most enzymes are much larger than the substrates they act on, and only a small portion of the protein (around three to four amino acids) is directly involved in catalysis. The region that contains these catalytic residues, binds the substrate, and then carries out the reaction is known as the *active site*. Enzymes can also contain sites that bind *cofactors*, non-protein molecules that are needed for catalysis.

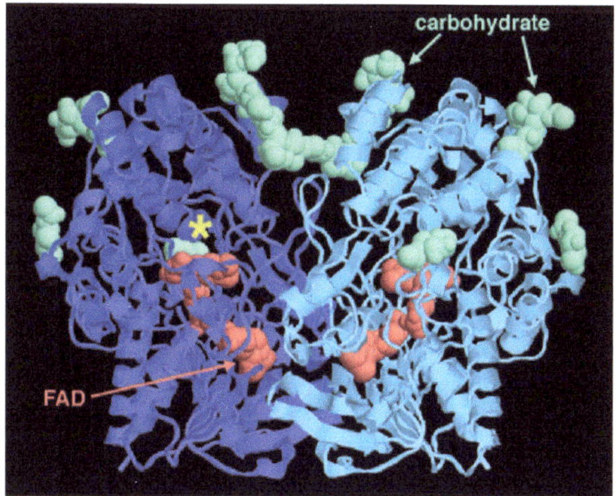

Fig. 2.5 Dimeric structure of GOD

Cofactors

Some enzymes do not need any additional component to show full activity. However, *others require non-protein molecules called cofactors to be bound for activity*. A cofactor is a non-protein chemical compound that is bound (either tightly or loosely) to an enzyme and is required for catalysis. Cofactors can be considered helper molecules/ions that assist in biochemical transformations. Certain substances such as water and various abundant ions may be bound tightly by enzymes but are not considered to be cofactors because they are ubiquitous and rarely limiting. Cofactors can be divided into two broad groups: prosthetic groups and coenzymes.

Prosthetic groups: *Permanent part* of the protein structure

Coenzymes: Small organic molecules that carry chemical groups between enzymes. These molecules are not bound tightly by the enzymes and are *released* as a normal part of the catalytic cycle

Examples of a prosthetic group and a coenzyme are, respectively, the flavin adenine dinucleotide (FAD) for GOD and the nicotinamide adenine dinucleotide (NAD^+) for GDH. An enzyme without its cofactor is referred to as an apoenzyme, while the completely active form (containing the cofactor) is called a holoenzyme:

$$\text{Apoenzyme} + \text{cofactor} \rightleftarrows \text{Holoenzyme}$$

For example, when applying denaturing conditions, the subunits of GOD dissociate with a concomitant loss of FAD.

Specificity

Enzymes are usually very specific as to which reactions they catalyse and the substrates that are involved in these reactions. The complementary shape, charge and hydrophilic/hydrophobic characteristics of enzymes and substrates are responsible for this specificity. The model that is currently most accepted to describe biocatalysis and enzyme/substrate/coenzyme interactions is referred to as the *induced fit model*. According to this model, the substrate does not simply bind to a rigid active site; in contrast, the amino acid side chains that make up the active site are moulded into the precise positions that enable the enzyme to perform its catalytic function. The active site continues to change until the substrate is completely bound, at which point the final shape and charge are determined.

Glucose quantitation is based on one of three enzymes: GOD, glucose-1-dehydrogenases (GDHs) or hexokinase [6].

Carbohydrate Chemistry

Glucose

β-D-glucose ($C_6H_{12}O_6$, molar mass 180.156 g mol^{-1}, also known as corn, grape or blood sugar) is one of the most important carbohydrates in biology since living cells use it as a source of energy and as a metabolic intermediate. In chemistry, glucose—a monosaccharide formed by six carbon atoms and containing an aldehyde functionality—is referred to as aldohexose. In solution, it undergoes the following equilibrium (Fig. 2.6):

The glucose molecule does exist in both an open-chain (acyclic) and a cyclic form; the cyclic one is, however, predominant in solution at pH 7. In solid phase, glucose only assumes the cyclic form.

Aldohexose sugars have four chiral centres yielding a total of $2^4 = 16$ stereoisomers. These are split into two groups, L and D isomers, with eight sugars in each. Only 7 of the 16 stereoisomers are found in living organisms, of which D-glucose, D-galactose and D-mannose are the most important.

When glucose cyclises into the ring structure, two additional isomers (or anomers) are obtained: α-glucose and β-glucose (Fig. 2.7). The anomers differ structurally by the relative positioning of the hydroxyl group linked to C-1. When

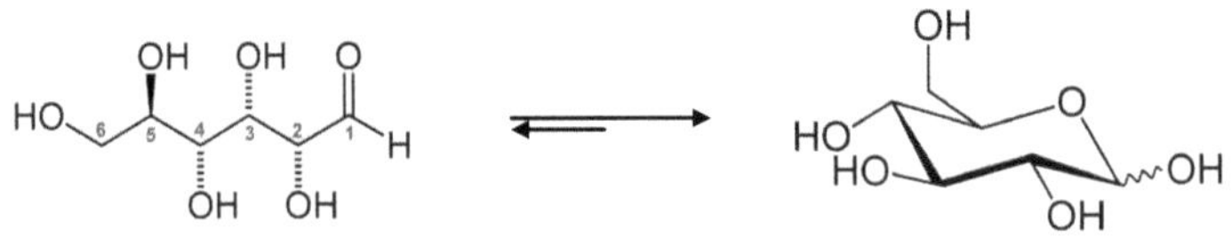

Fig. 2.6 Equilibrium between acyclic and cyclic forms of glucose

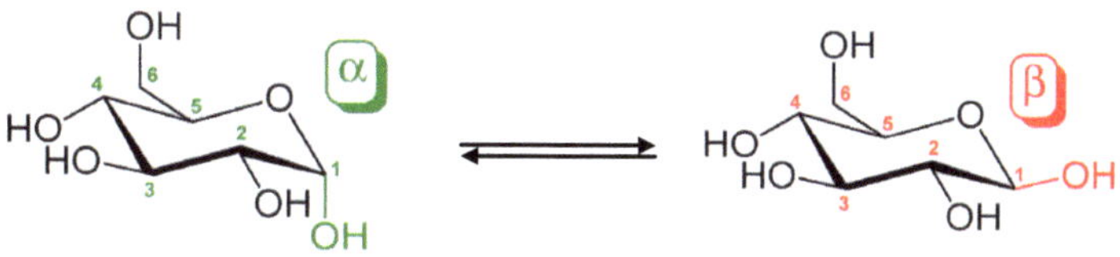

Fig. 2.7 Mutarotation equilibrium: α- (*left*) and β- (*right*) glucose

Fig. 2.8 Maltose chemical structure

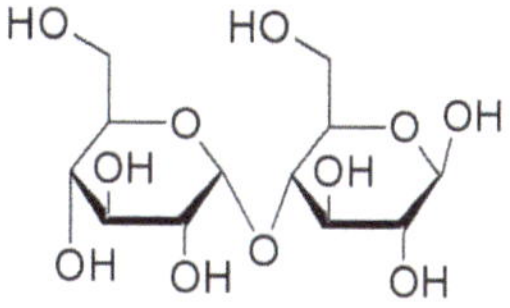

dissolving solid glucose in an aqueous medium, the α and β forms interconvert over a time scale of hours in a process called mutarotation. The final and stable α:β ratio is 36 : 64.

Interfering Sugars

Sugars other than glucose are normally found in the blood at very low concentrations. There are, however, specific pathological or clinical cases in which their blood concentration can be unusually high, and these molecules become important sources of interference. As a result, glycaemic levels are typically overestimated.

Maltose

Maltose is a disaccharide formed from two units of glucose joined together (Fig. 2.8).

Although maltose is not normally present in the human body, its blood concentration can be relevant in the following cases:

- When intravenous drips are administered (e.g. cases in which water/energy must be supplied parenterally);
- In cases where peritoneal dialysis solution containing icodextrin is administered. Icodextrin (EXTRANEAL, Baxter Healthcare Corporation Deerfield, IL 60015 USA) is a polymer of maltose that breaks down into maltose in the human body.

Xylose

Xylose (Fig. 2.9a) is a monosaccharide present in the human body at concentrations normally much lower than that of glucose (a few milligrams per decilitre only).

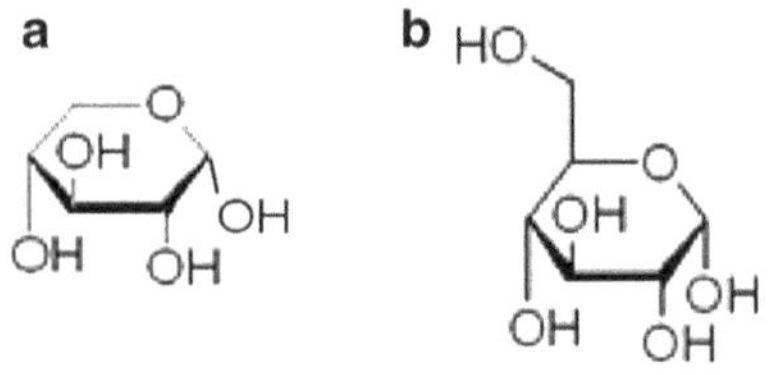

Fig. 2.9 Xylose (**a**) versus glucose (**b**) chemical structures

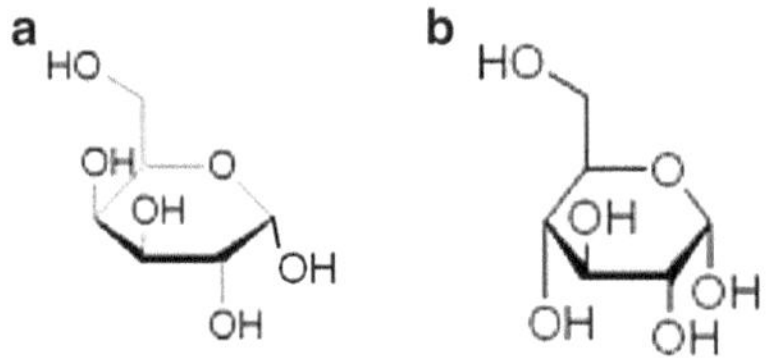

Fig. 2.10 Galactose (**a**) versus glucose (**b**) chemical structures

However, its concentration can increase when xylose absorption tests are carried out. Such tests are performed to determine whether or not digestive and absorptive processes are normally proceeding in the intestinal canal.

Galactose

Galactose (Fig. 2.10a) is a monosaccharide that, after absorption and transportation to the liver, is converted onto glucose for use as energy.

Thus, galactose is normally present in the peripheral blood at very low concentrations (less than 1 mg/dL). The amount of such sugar dissolved in the blood can, however, increase due to the following diseases:

- Deficiency of metabolic enzyme in the liver (congenital metabolic abnormality)
- Decline of metabolic function caused by hepatocellular damage from viral hepatitis and other diseases
- Decline of effective hepatic blood flow caused by liver cirrhosis and other diseases
- Galactose levels increase when galactose tolerance tests are carried out.

Other Sugars

Sugars other than the aforementioned ones are also normally checked as possible interferents. These can include fructose, mannose and lactose but also alcohol sugars such as mannitol and xylitol (Fig. 2.11). Their interfering action is, however, typically low.

Mannitol is a sugar alcohol, that is, it is derived from a sugar by reduction. Mannitol is also used as a sweetener for people with diabetes. Since mannitol has a positive heat of solution, it is used as a sweetener in breath-freshening candies and chewing gums.

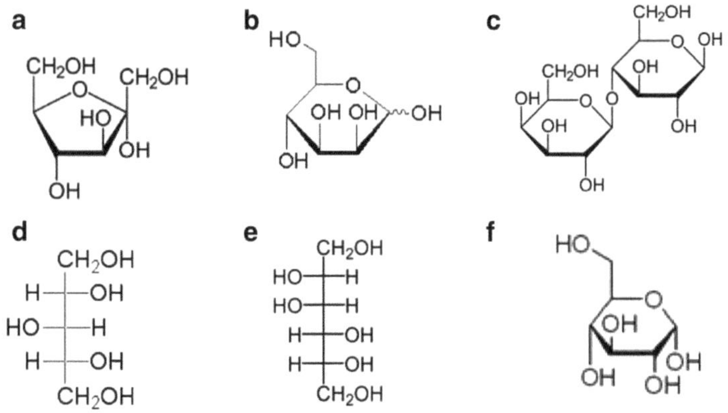

Fig. 2.11 Fructose (**a**), mannose (**b**), lactose (**c**), xylitol (**d**), mannitol (**e**) versus glucose (**f**) chemical structures

Xylitol is a sugar alcohol roughly as sweet as sucrose with only two-thirds the food energy. Possessing approximately 40% less food energy, xylitol is a low-calorie alternative to table sugar. Absorbed more slowly than sugar, it does not contribute to high blood sugar levels or the resulting hyperglycaemia caused by insufficient insulin response.

Glucose Oxidase (GOD or GOx)

GOD is the enzyme that catalyses the oxidation of β-D-glucose into D-glucono-1,5-lactone and hydrogen peroxide (H_2O_2) using molecular oxygen (O_2) as the electron acceptor. D-glucono-1,5-lactone subsequently hydrolyses to gluconic acid (Fig. 2.12).

When produced commercially for biosensing applications, GOD is often extracted from the fungus *Aspergillus niger*. GOD from *A. niger* is a dimer of two identical subunits held together by disulphide bonds [7, 8] (Fig. 2.13a). Each subunit also contains a flavin adenine dinucleotide (FAD) cofactor (Fig. 2.13b), not covalently but tightly bound at specific sites of such macromolecules [9] (Fig. 2.13c). When bound, FAD helps stabilise the three-dimensional structure of the macromolecule.

Specific information (mainly from Ref. [8]):

- A GOD holoenzyme is made up of two identical subunits, each with a molecular weight of 80 kDa (160 kDa for the whole enzyme).
- Each monomer contains a tightly bound ($K = 1 \times 10^{-10}$) FAD cofactor (Fig. 2.10b). Strong denaturing conditions are needed to induce the release of such prosthetic groups from the holoprotein.
- FAD might be replaceable with FHD (flavin-hypoxanthine dinucleotide) without loss of activity.

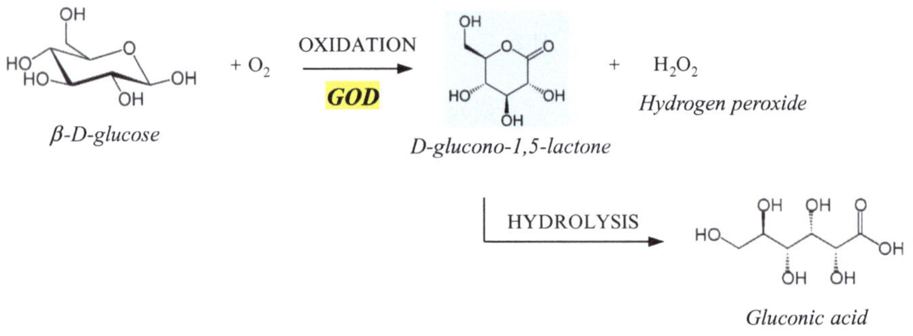

β-D-glucose + O_2 OXIDATION GOD → D-glucono-1,5-lactone + H_2O_2 Hydrogen peroxide

HYDROLYSIS → Gluconic acid

Fig. 2.12 GOD-mediated oxidation of glucose

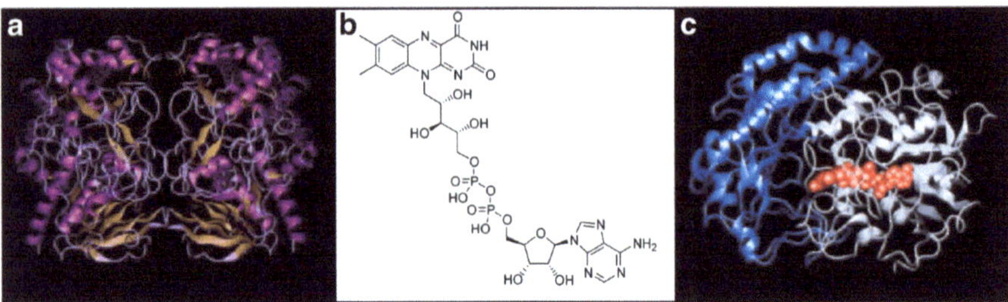

Fig. 2.13 (**a**) Overall topology of GOD holoenzyme; (**b**) molecular structure of FAD cofactor; (**c**) subunit structure of GOD showing FAD (*red* spacefill)

- The enzyme is glycosylated, having a carbohydrate content of approximately 16–20% (w/w).
- The total dimensions of the dimer are 70 × 55 × 80 Ångstroms [$1\ \text{Å} = 10^{-10}$ m].
- The native protein is acidic, having an isoelectric point (pI) of 4.2.
- GOD shows catalytic activity over pH values that range from 3 to 10 (the optimum being pH = 5.5).
- Literature values for the Michaelis-Menten constant of GOD are approximately 15–20 mM for glucose [8] and 0.2 mM for molecular oxygen [10] (which can be seen as the second substrate).
- In the electrochemically relevant half-reaction in which glucose is oxidised by GOD, approximately 5×10^3 glucose molecules are oxidised per second [11].

Some differences in the foregoing parameters can, however, be observed if using GODs obtained from sources other than *A. niger*. It should be noted that enzymes extracted from different organisms might differ slightly in their amino acid sequence. Although infrequent, whenever these changes involve the residues of the active site, the degree of specificity of the enzyme toward different carbohydrates can obviously change. Scientists have recently employed the most advanced techniques of site-directed mutagenesis (i.e. genetic engineering) to improve the characteristics of glucose-reacting enzymes. Pertinent examples are the efforts to enhance both thermal stability and substrate specificity of GDHs [12].

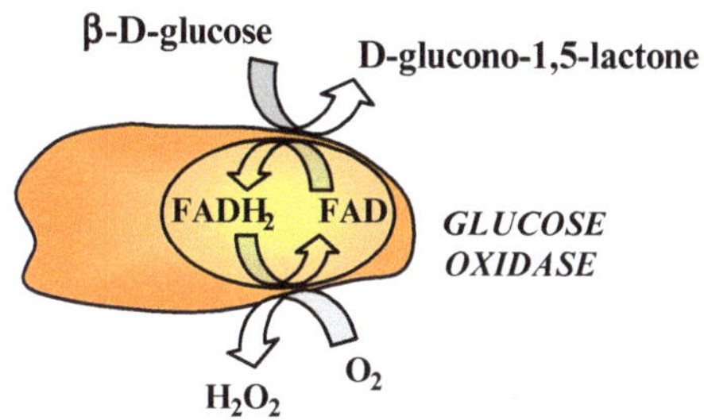

Fig. 2.14 GOD-mediated biocatalytic oxidation of glucose. The active site of the enzyme (containing FAD as the prosthetic group) is indicated as a "cavity" in this scheme

GOD-Mediated Oxidation of Glucose: Mechanism

To make GOD work as a catalyst (Fig. 2.14), the presence of the FAD prosthetic group is essential. Indeed, in the GOD-catalysed oxidation of glucose, FAD works as the initial electron acceptor and is reduced to $FADH_2$. $FADH_2$ is then oxidised back to FAD by the final electron acceptor, molecular oxygen. Accepting electrons from $FADH_2$, O_2 is finally reduced to hydrogen peroxide (H_2O_2).

The overall reaction is a cascade of redox processes in which the electrons flow from the redox couple with the lowest reduction potential (i.e. the gluconolactone/glucose pair, E'°= −0.320 V versus SHE [13]) to the couple with the highest reduction potential (i.e. the H_2O_2/O_2 pair, E'°= +0.290 V versus SHE) through the intermediate one (i.e. the enzyme cofactor, $FADH_2$/FAD pair, E'°= +0.030 V versus SHE [14]):

$$C_6H_{12}O_6 \longrightarrow C_6H_{10}O_6 + 2\,H^+ + 2e^- \qquad E'^\circ = -0.320\ V$$

$$FAD + 2H^+ + 2e^- \rightleftarrows FADH_2 \qquad E'^\circ = +0.030\ V$$

$$O_2 + 2H^+ + 2e^- \longrightarrow H_2O_2 \qquad E'^\circ = +0.290\ V$$

$$\underline{C_6H_{12}O_6 + O_2 \longrightarrow C_6H_{10}O_6 + H_2O_2\ (\text{net reaction})}$$

where E'° indicates the apparent formal redox potential of the different redox couples and SHE stands for standard hydrogen electrode, the reference electrode against which the formal potential of all the other redox couples is evaluated. The formal redox potential (E°') expresses the tendency of a chemical species to accept or donate electrons. The more positive the redox potential, the higher this tendency to steal electrons from other species.

The chemical structure and detailed redox chemistry of the FAD cofactor are presented in Fig. 2.15.

Radio-labelled O_2 and water have been used to show that the oxygen in hydrogen peroxide (product of the reaction) only derives from the gaseous O_2 dissolved in the glucose sample, rather than water itself. In nature, O_2 is the essential cosubstrate of GOD. However, the role of oxygen could drastically change depending on

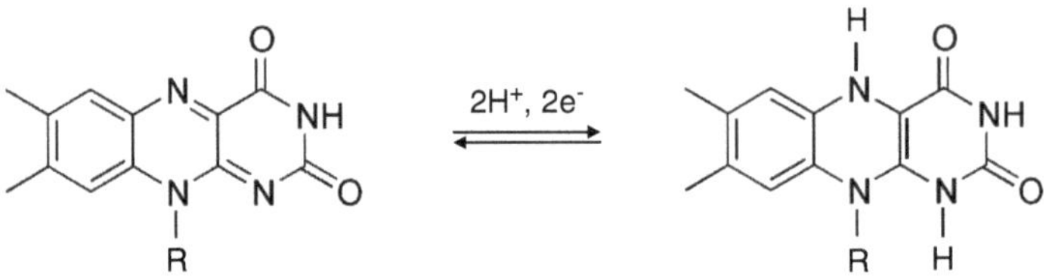

Fig. 2.15 Redox chemistry of FAD cofactor

Table 2.3 Relative GOD-catalysed oxidation rates for different sugars [8]; these rates are normalised to the rate observed for β-D-glucose and for the general reaction: sugar + O_2 → corresponding acid + H_2O_2

Sugar	Relative oxidation rate
β-D-glucose	100
α-D-glucose	0.64
D-mannose	0.98
D-xylose	0.98
Tetralose	0.28
Maltose	0.19
Galactose	0.14
Melobiose	0.11

which bioelectrochemical strategy the test strip adopts to sense blood glucose concentrations [15]. How different levels of oxygenation of a sample affect the quality of glucose measurements will be further discussed where appropriate.

Specificity of GOD

The enzyme is highly specific for β-D-glucose. The α-anomer and the other sugars are practically not acted upon (Table 2.3).

Glucose 1-Dehydrogenase (GDH)

GDHs form a class of enzymes relatively less cofactor- and substrate-specific than GOD. On one hand, GOD only admits FAD as its prosthetic group and reacts essentially with β-D-glucose. On the other hand, different members of the GDH family can use different cofactors [i.e. nicotinamide adenine dinucleotide (NAD^+) or nicotinamide adenine dinucleotide phosphate ($NADP^+$), ubiquinone (coenzyme Q_{10}), pyrroloquinoline quinone (PQQ) and FAD] (Fig. 2.16) and often show significant cross-reactivity with carbohydrates other than glucose:

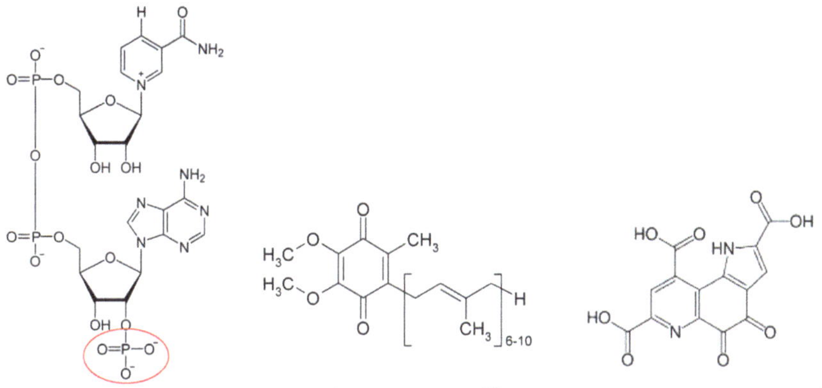

NAD(P)$^{+}$ (E′° = - 0.324 V)[15] **Ubiquinone** (E′° = + 0.045 V)[15]

PQQ (E′° = +0.010 V)[11]

Fig. 2.16 Molecular structure and redox potentials (versus SHE at 25°C and pH 7) of NADP^{+}, ubiquinone and PQQ. NADP^{+} is distinguished from NAD^{+} by the phosphate functionality, which is highlighted in *red*

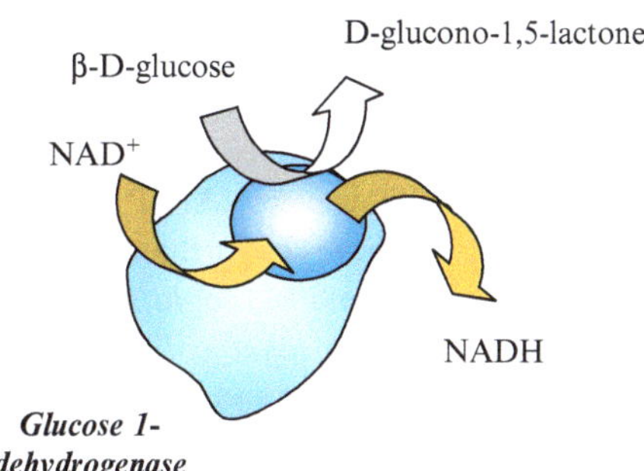

Fig. 2.17 Biocatalytic oxidation of glucose mediated by a NAD^{+}-dependent GDH. The active site of the enzyme (where NAD^{+} is reduced and glucose oxidised) is indicated in *blue*

GDH-Mediated Oxidation of Glucose: Mechanism

Independently of the employed cofactor (and similarly to GOD), GDHs also oxidise glucose to D-glucono-1,5-lactone. As a major advantage of these reactions over those catalysed by GOD, the former do not require the presence of molecular oxygen. For example, the reaction for a GDH NAD(P)$^{+}$-dependent is

$$\beta\text{-D-glucose} + \text{NAD(P)}^{+} \rightleftarrows \text{D-glucono-1,5-lactone} + \text{NAD(P)H} + \text{H}^{+}$$

This reaction is schematically depicted in Fig. 2.17.

This enzyme admits either NAD^{+} or NADP^{+} as the electron acceptor. Since NAD^{+} and NADP^{+} are released during the catalytic cycle, they can be classified as coenzymes of GDH (in contrast to FAD and PQQ, which are tightly bound prosthetic groups).

The dehydrogenases that use either ubiquinone or PQQ as their cofactor are classified as quinoprotein GDHs. In bacteria that produce the apoenzyme, the latter can be easily reconstituted into an active holoenzyme by adding PQQ and a metal ion (such as Ca^{2+}) to the medium [16]. Both PQQ and Ca^{2+} are firmly bound to the protein. The resulting PQQ enzyme can exhibit catalytic activities up to 20 times higher than that of GOD [17].

Specific information (mainly from Ref. [17]):

- GDH from *B. subtilis* (EC 1.1.1.47) is a homotetrameric protein with a molecular weight of 126 kDa.
- This enzyme employs $NAD(P)^+$ as its cofactor.
- The enzyme shows a pH optimum at 8.0 and a temperature optimum at 25°C.
- The literature values for the Michaelis-Menten constant of this GDH are in the range 5–55 mM for β-D-glucose and 0.1–0.3 mM for $NAD(P)^+$, depending on the exact experimental conditions.
- The pI of the protein is 4.8.

Specificity of GDHs

As for GOD, GDHs only react with the β-anomer of glucose (being inactive on α-D-glucose). However, $NAD(P)^+$-dependent GDH also shows substantial activity toward carbohydrates other than glucose (including D-xylose and galactose). GDH from *Thermoplasma acidophilum* (Sigma-Aldrich, St Louis, MO, recombinant, expressed in *Escherichia coli*) shows, for example, an activity $\geq$100 units/mg protein toward glucose and $\geq$50 units/mg protein toward galactose.

Since oxygen is not involved in the reaction pathway of GDHs, GDH-based blood glucose meters have the advantage of being free from the influence of dissolved oxygen. However, as compared to GOD, $NAD(P)^+$-dependent GDHs typically suffer from poor stability and require the addition of a coenzyme. In addition, PQQ-dependent enzymes have the drawback of possessing poor substrate specificity and reacting to saccharides other than glucose (e.g. maltose and lactose), thereby deteriorating the accuracy of the measurements. A sensor based on PQQ-GDHs may overestimate the glucose concentration in a blood sample containing such saccharides. Recently (August 2009), the US Food and Drug Administration (FDA), for example, released a Public Health Notification to alert healthcare practitioners about the possibility of fatal clinical errors associated with the use of GDH/PQQ-based glucose monitoring systems.

Among the different members of the GDH family, the flavin-bound GDH (FAD-GDH) isolated from *Aspergillus terreus* [10] represents an exception, having demonstrated thermostability, a large Michaelis constant for glucose and a superior substrate specificity (Table 2.4).

This FAD-dependent GDH combines the oxygen independence of PQQ-GDH with the specificity (toward non-glucose sugars) of GOD. Significant cross-reaction

Table 2.4 Relative substrate specificity of GOD and NAD^+-, PQQ- and FAD-dependent GDHs [10, 18, 19]

Substrate	GOD	NAD^+-dependent GDH	PQQ-dependent GDH	FAD-dependent GDH
D-Glucose	100	100	100	100
D-Xylose	1	n.a.	n.a.	9
D-Galactose	10	0	12–15	0
D-Mannose	13	10	17	2
Maltose	10	0	71–98	2
Sucrose	10	0	0	n.a.
Fructose	10	0	0	n.a.
Lactose	10	1	56	0

n.a. not applicable

is only observed in the case of D-xylose; use of this sugar, even in clinical settings, is, however, extremely rare [20].

Moreover, in contrast to PQQ-GDHs, FAD-GDH is not inhibited by EDTA because its activity is independent of the presence of Ca^{2+} or Mg^{2+}. Its ever wider use in the development of glucosensors can therefore be easily envisioned.

Electrochemical Sensing of Glucose

Different electrochemical glucose sensors may strongly vary in their signal transduction mode. These can be loosely classified as follows:

(I) Mediator-less systems, where the electrical response arises from the oxidation of the natural product of the enzymatic reaction (i.e. hydrogen peroxide, H_2O_2);
(II) Mediator-assisted systems, where electrons are transported from the active site of the enzyme to the electrode surface with the aid of a redox reagent;
(III) Systems based on direct electron transfer, where the electrons derived from glucose oxidation directly flow from the active site of the enzyme to the electrode surface.

Particularly relevant for the purposes of this document are the first and second classes of sensor.

Mediator-less Glucosensors (GOD-Based Systems Only)

These glucosensors rely on the direct detection of the H_2O_2 generated by GOD through the reaction depicted in Fig. 2.18. While oxidising glucose, the prosthetic group of the enzyme (FAD) is reduced to $FADH_2$. The oxidised form of the

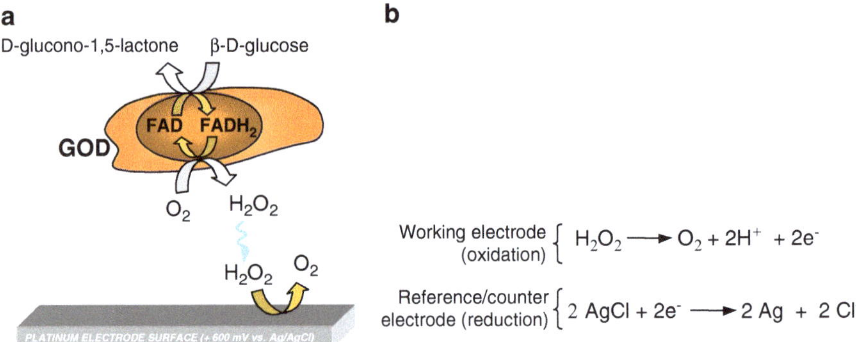

Fig. 2.18 (**a**) Electrochemical oxidation of H_2O_2 at platinum electrodes. (**b**) Complete balance of reactions occurring at both working and reference/counter electrodes during H_2O_2 detection

cofactor is then regenerated via electron transfer to the natural electron acceptor of GOD (i.e. molecular oxygen, O_2). As a result, hydrogen peroxide is produced. It is important to stress here that *regeneration of the oxidised form of FAD is essential for the establishment of biocatalysis*. In the absence of electron acceptors GOD could not further process additional glucose molecules! In these glucosensors, H_2O_2 is typically detected by poising a platinum (Pt) electrode at a fixed oxidising potential (i.e. + 600 mV versus Ag/AgCl—Fig. 2.18).

An electrical signal is produced following electron transfer from the peroxide to the Pt electrode; such an enzyme-catalysed current is, under suitable conditions, proportional to glucose concentration.

Examples of systems that work according to this principle are both the GlucoDay S and the Yellow Springs (YSI) glucose analysers.

Mediator-Assisted Glucosensors (GOD- and GDH-Based Systems)

As will be discussed in section "Oxygen Limitation", mediator-less systems may suffer from limited accuracy whenever O_2 represents a limiting reagent (i.e. in hypoxemic patients or at very high glycaemic levels). This problem was circumvented with the development of mediator-assisted glucosensors.

As a result of their reaction with glucose, both GODs and GDHs are brought into a reduced (electron-rich) state. Hence, re-oxidation of the cofactor in their active site is a crucial step before the enzymes can process further glucose molecules. Similarly to other redox enzymes, the active sites of GODs and GDHs tend to reside within clefts or folds within the macromolecular structure of the protein. As a consequence, the thick polypeptidic layer that surrounds the redox centre does not normally allow for the direct transfer of electrons to conventional electrodes. This electron transfer

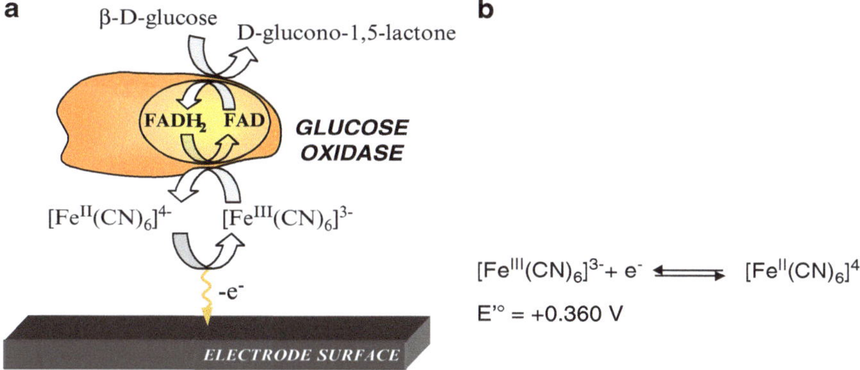

Fig. 2.19 (**a**) GOD-based glucosensor: mediator-assisted bioelectrochemical oxidation of glucose. (**b**) Ferri-/ferro-cyanide redox chemistry

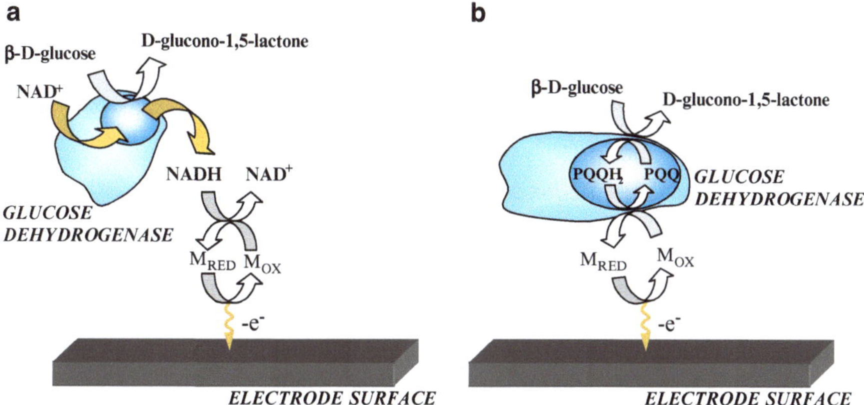

Fig. 2.20 Mediator-assisted bioelectrochemical oxidation of glucose using a GDH-based glucosensor. (**a**) NAD^+- and (**b**) PQQ-dependent glucose dehydrogenases

may be, however, facilitated by inclusion of an electron carrier or mediator, a chemical species capable of shuttling electrons from the redox centre of the enzyme to the surface of the electrode. The oxidised form of the mediator takes up electrons from the reduced cofactor and then, in the reduced state, transports them to the electrode, where it becomes re-oxidised (e.g. Fig. 2.19).

Similar arguments are also valid for GDH-based glucosensors. Figure 2.20 schematically shows the working principle of both $NAD(P)^+$ and PQQ-dependent GDHs. In both cases, use of a redox mediator (M_{OX}) is necessary to lower the overvoltage required for oxidising the enzyme cofactor.

Although O_2 is not a cosubstrate for GDHs, and much lower glucose concentrations can be detected using this enzyme, some O_2 may still be reduced at the potentials at which the GDH electrodes are poised [21]. Clearly, this kind

Table 2.5 Key features of selected electrochemical test strips

Strip	Electrodic material	Mediator	Enzyme	Enzyme cofactor
OneTouch Vita	Graphite	Potassium ferricyanide	GOD	FAD
GlucoMen Visio V1	Graphite	Hexaammine ruthenium (III) chloride	GOD	FAD
GLUCOCARD G sensor	Graphite	Potassium ferricyanide	GDH	FAD
Ascensia Contour	—	Potassium ferricyanide	GDH	FAD
GLUCOFIX sensor	Gold	Potassium ferricyanide	GOD	FAD
GlucoMen LX sensor	Gold	Potassium ferricyanide	GOD	FAD
FreeStyle lite	Graphite	Polymeric Os (III) complex	GDH	PQQ
Precision Xtra	—	Phenanthroline quinone	GDH	NAD^+
Accu-Check Aviva	Gold	Nitrosoaniline[a]	GDH	PQQ

[a] Activated to quinonediimine

of interference would be particularly relevant at very low glucose concentrations, where the glucose-dependent component of the current recorded by the meter is comparable to the background signal.

Criteria for Choosing a Redox Mediator

Considerations in mediator choice include redox potential, stability in mixtures with proteins, solubility and rate of dissolution, cost and intellectual property rights. Potassium ferricyanide, $K_3[Fe^{III}(CN)_6]$, is one of the most widely employed mediators in the electrochemical test strips currently on the market. As exemplified by Table 2.5, several other options are, however, available.

Irrespectively of its inorganic or organic nature, the mediator must generate a reversible redox couple. This means that the molecule must be capable of rapidly exchanging electrons with both electron donors (i.e. reducing compounds), acceptors (i.e. oxidising compounds) and, of course, electrodes. Such reversible redox couples are also often referred to as fast mediators.

The biological samples in which glucose must be measured often also contain a number of endogenous or exogenous chemicals that are themselves electroactive. In many cases, however, oxidation of these compounds requires the application of relatively high potentials. Hence, the second criterion that guides the choice of mediator is its redox potential. On one hand, it must be sufficiently high to allow easy extraction of electrons from the reduced form of the enzyme cofactor (whatever it is). On the other hand, re-oxidation of the reduced form of the mediator at the electrode surface must be achieved at relatively low potentials (preferably $<+0.4$ V versus Ag/AgCl), where the non-specific oxidation rate of the interfering endogenous/exogenous compounds is negligible.

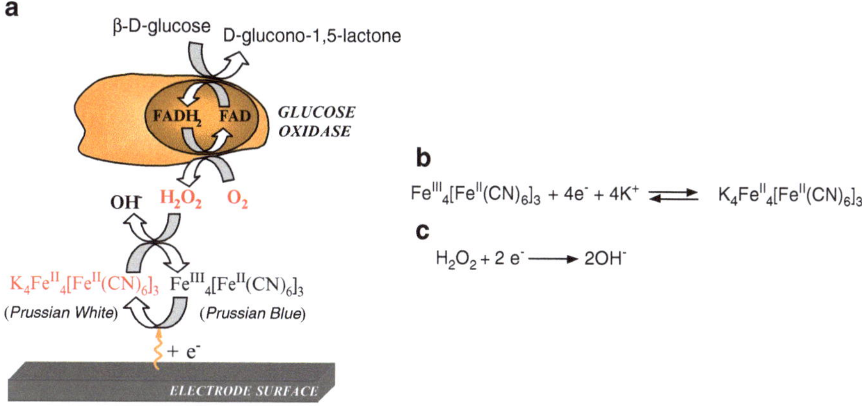

Fig. 2.21 (**a**) Overall bioelectrochemical reactions occurring at surface of GlucoMen Day sensor. (**b**) Prussian Blue/Prussian White redox chemistry. (**c**) Reduction of hydrogen peroxide to hydroxyl ion

The mediating redox couple can be freely diffusing, directly bound to GOD (e.g. via a short spacer arm) or bound to a highly cross-linked GOD-entrapping hydrogel. For freely diffusing mediators, solubility and fast dissolution of the salt are crucial. Indeed, as the fastest assays are now completed in 4 to 5 s, the mediator must dissolve into the applied blood sample in 1 s or less.

Hybrid Glucosensors

Herein, the term hybrid is used to indicate glucose biosensors that combine features that are characteristic of (GOD-based) mediator-less systems with features that, in contrast, recall mediated glucosensors. This is specifically the case with the technology implemented in the glucose biosensor of GlucoMen Day. The carbon working electrode surface of the GlucoMen Day sensor is modified with an atypical redox mediator, the ferric hexacyanoferrate or Prussian Blue. Being insoluble in aqueous media, this chemical does not shuttle electrons from the active site of the enzyme to the electrode surface (like all other mediators) but rather exerts an electrocatalytic activity towards H_2O_2, the product generated by the surface-immobilised GOD (Fig. 2.21).

Electrocatalytic reduction of hydrogen peroxide to hydroxyl ions is achieved at very low potentials (approximately 0.0 V versus Ag/AgCl) where most of the common endogenous and exogenous species (including ascorbic acid and paracetamol) do not yet interfere.

Interferents on Blood Glucose Quantitation

Accuracy (and precision) of blood glucose quantitation can be affected by a number of physical (environmental) and (bio)chemical factors. The compounds known to act as interferents can be broadly divided into two groups (Table 2.6): endogenous substances (i.e. related to physio-pathological conditions of the patient) and exogenous substances (i.e. drugs).

Table 2.7 presents a comprehensive list of drugs [22] that may be checked as possible interferents of blood glucose monitoring systems. Note that for each drug the test level suggested by the National Committee for Clinical Laboratory Standards (NCCLS) is calculated as 10 times the therapeutic dose.

Table 2.8 also reports a list of suggested standard interferents developed by the FDA (interferents at concentrations 10 times higher than the therapeutic dose) also obtained from NCCLS [23].

Biosensors are typically tested at two glucose concentrations (low and high), with and without interferent, to determine the possible signal variation associated with the presence of a non-glucose species. Generally, a response deviation of less than ±15 mg/dL or ±20% is considered acceptable. This clearly does not mean that the species does not interfere at all!

The chemical structure of some endogenous and exogenous interfering chemicals is reported in Fig. 2.22:

The interferences can be at different levels of the biosensor architecture: enzyme, mediator, and electrode. Table 2.9 summarises the most common sources of interferences.

Interferents Acting at the Enzyme Level

Cross-Reactivity with Sugars Other Than Glucose

Each enzyme recognises specific functional groups of its substrate. This is clearly true also in the case of GODs and GDHs. Figure 2.23, for example, schematically represents the interactions established by β-D-glucose at the active site of the GOD expressed by *Penicillium amagasakiense*. This active site exposes several amino acidic residues (tyrosine 73, phenylalanine 418, tryptophan 430, arginine 516, asparagine 518 and histidines 520 and 563) which, along with the FAD cofactor, establish hydrogen bonds and hydrophobic interactions with glucose.

Table 2.6 Types of interfering substances acting at enzyme level

Endogenous substances	Haematocrit, haemoglobin, bilirubin, uric acid, lipids, proteins, O_2 ......
Exogenous substances	Ascorbic acid, paracetamol, dopamine, maltose, mannitol .....

Table 2.7 Therapeutic, toxic and recommended test concentrations for several drugs

Generic name	Therapeutic level	Toxic level	Test level NCCLS	1	2	3
Acetaminophen	10–20	150	200	200[b]	300	1,000
Acetylsalicylic acid	20–100	150–300	500	500[b]	450	3,000
Aminophylline	10–20	30–40	250	250[b]	240	40
Ampicillin	5	NA	50	50[b]	2,500	3,750
Ascorbic acid	8–12	NA	30	30[b]	240	300
Cefazolin	400	NA	4,000	4,000[b]	3,200	8,000
Cimetidine	1–10	NA	100	100[b]	7	14
Dexamethasone	NA	NA	NA	4[c]	20	60
Digoxin	>0.0008	0.0017–0.0033	NA	0.0033[d]	0.003	0.08
Dobutamine	35–50	NA	NA	0.5	0.05	NA
Dopamine	NA	NA	130	130[b]	60	NA
Epinephrine	NA	NA	NA	0.2[c]	0.7	1.4
Erythromycin	2–20	NA	200	200[b]	NA	NA
Furosemide	1–3	NA	20	20[b]	30	60
Gentamicin	8–12	10–30	120	120[b]	30	NA
Glipizide	NA	NA	NA	4[c]	18	24
Heparin sodium	NA	NA	8	8[b]	94	105
Hydralazine	0.1	NA	NA	1[d]	NA	NA
Lidocaine	1.5–6	9–14	60	60[b]	120	NA
Mannitol	NA	NA	NA	20,000[e]	24,000	NA
Nitroglycerin	0.0012–0.011	NA	NA	0.11[d]	0.1	0.3
Nitroprusside	NA	NA	NA	7.5[c]	12	NA
Norepinephrine	NA	NA	NA	10[e]	15	NA
Penicillin G potassium	NA	NA	NA	2,400[e]	7,000	NA
Phentolamine	NA	NA	NA	5[e]	10	15
Phenytoin	10–20	20–40+	100	100[b]	NA	NA
Procainamide	4–10	10–12+	100	100[b]	40	20
Quinidine	0.3–6	10	50	50[b]	60	76
Regular insulin	100 or less	NA	NA	1,000[d]	200	50
Warfarin	1–10	NA	100	100[b]	180	NA

NA not available, *NCCLS* National Committee for Clinical Laboratory Standards

[a]Drug concentrations are expressed as micrograms per millilitre, except heparin sodium (units per millilitre) and regular insulin (microunits per millilitre). Dodutamine therapeutic levels were incorrect in *Goodman & Gilman's The Pharmacological Basis of Therapeutic* [8] and were taken from Steinberg and Notterman [7].

[b]Test level recommended by the National Committee for Clinical Laboratory Standards (NCCLS) [10].

[c]Estimated by distributing the highest dose published in *Goodman & Gilman's The Pharmacological Basis of Therapeutic* [8] in 5 L of blood volume. See "Methods and Materials."

[d]Toxic level or ten times the therapeutic level published in *Goodman & Gilman's The Pharmacological Basis of Therapeutic* [8].

[e]Estimated by distributing the highest dose published in *The Critical Care Drug Handbook* [9] in 5 L of blood volume.

Table 2.8 List of potential electrochemical interferents [11]

Interferent	Suggested test level (mg/dL)
Acetaminophen	20
Salicylic acid	50
Tetracycline	4
Dopamine	13
Ephedrine	10
Ibuprofen	40
l-DOPA	5
Methyl-DOPA	2.5
Tolazamide	100
Tolbutamide	100
Ascorbic acid	3
Bilirubin (unconjugated)	20
Cholesterol	500
Creatinine	30
Triglycerides	3,000
Urate	20

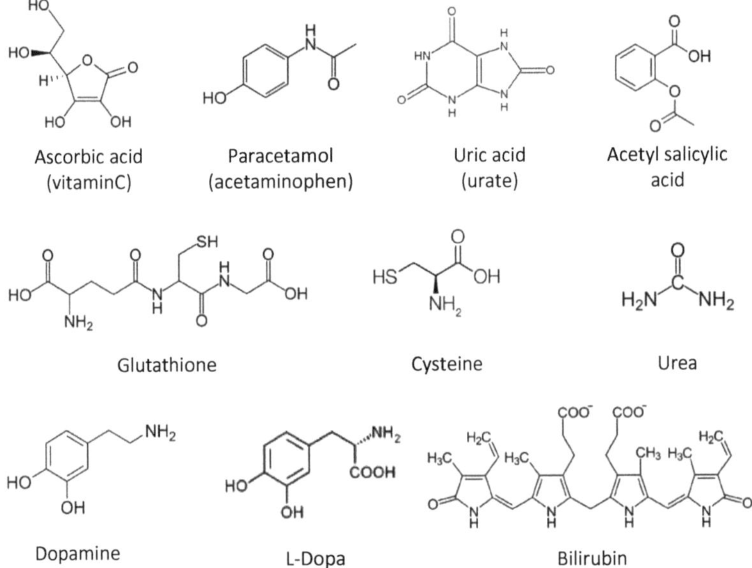

Fig. 2.22 Chemical structure of various interferents

Sugars that share strong similarities with the molecular structure of glucose can be erroneously recognised by the enzyme, thus leading to a non-specific enzymatic activity. In a glucosensor this directly translates into an overestimation of the glycaemic readings.

Table 2.9 Common interferents for each level of glucosensor architecture

Enzyme
Cross-reaction with sugars other than glucose
Oxygen limitation
Reducing chemicals
Extremes in pH
Redox mediator
Humidity
Oxygen
Generic reducing/oxidising compounds
Electrode surface
Surface 'fouling' (e.g. by lipids, haematocrit)
Oxidation/reduction of compounds with intrinsic electrochemical activity

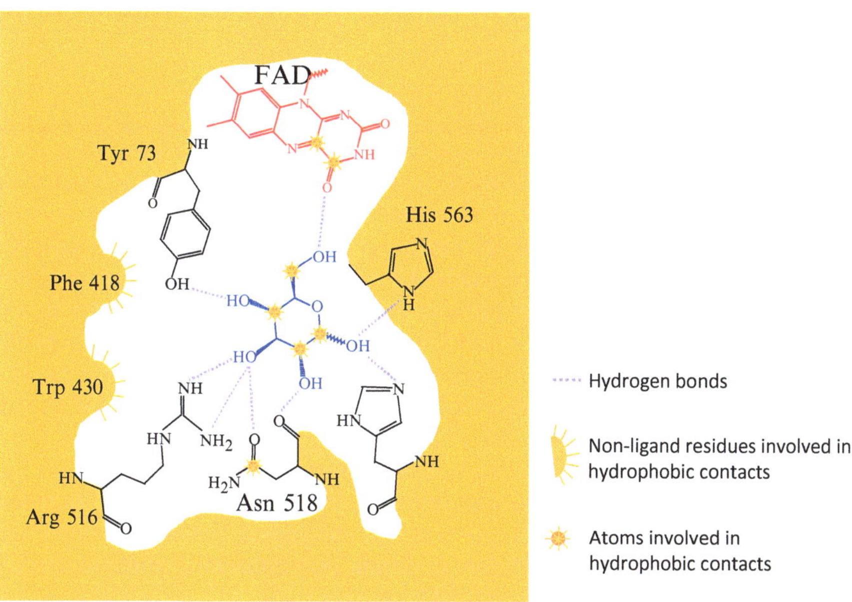

Fig. 2.23 Modelled interactions of β-D-glucose with active site residues in wild-type *P. amagasakiense* GOD [24]

The amino acidic residues of the active site can differ even in enzymes of the same family if these are expressed by different organisms. Taking into account that a variety of cofactors can additionally be bound, it is not surprising that the members of the GDH family exhibit a different ability to discriminate against non-glucose sugars.

The relative substrate specificity of the different glucose-processing enzymes is reported in Table 2.10. From those data, it clearly emerged that, although the

Table 2.10 Qualitative comparison: GOD versus FAD-dependent GDH

	Specificity	Turnover rate	Dependence on dissolved O_2	Stability
GOD	+++	++	Yes	+++
FAD-dependent GDH	++	+++	no	++

specificity of GOD is still unsurpassed, the FAD-GDH enzyme compares favourably with GOD. The characteristics of the two most suitable enzymes for the production of glucose biosensors are further qualitatively compared in Table 2.10.

Oxygen Limitation

According to the scheme

$$\text{Glucose} + O_2 \xrightarrow{GOD} \text{Gluconolactone} + H_2O_2$$

glucose and oxygen (substrate and cosubstrate of GOD, respectively) must react at a 1:1 stoichiometric ratio. However, it is important to take into account their different water solubilities. While the concentration of glucose in an undiluted blood sample can be as high as 30 mM, the saturating concentration of O_2 in an aqueous medium at 25°C is only approximately 0.2 mM (i.e. 150 times lower). For this reason, mediator-less systems are prone to underestimate blood glucose readings if used on hypoxemic patients ($pO_2 < 55$ mmHg). This problem can be particularly relevant when the blood sugar levels are very high and oxygen seriously represents a limiting reagent. In these cases, the response of a blood glucose meter would rapidly deviate from linearity, as shown in Fig. 2.24.

The environmental conditions and physio-pathological states that can lead to abnormally low blood oxygen concentrations include living at high altitudes, acute conditions (asthma, pulmonary oedema, pneumonia, pulmonary embolism, pneumothorax) and chronic conditions (anaemia, polycythaemia, emphysema, pulmonary fibrosis, lung neoplasm, cerebral lesions).

Reducing Chemicals

In mediator-less systems, the H_2O_2 generated by GOD should only react at the electrode surface in order to generate a current that is directly proportional to the original glucose concentration. However, if the blood sample contains reducing chemicals such as ascorbic acid or acetaminophen, these compounds can consume the peroxide through a parasite reaction (Fig. 2.25). The blood glucose levels are, consequently, underestimated. The impact of this interference could probably be mitigated by shortening the time needed to complete the blood test. However, to our knowledge there are no systems currently capable of completely compensating for it.

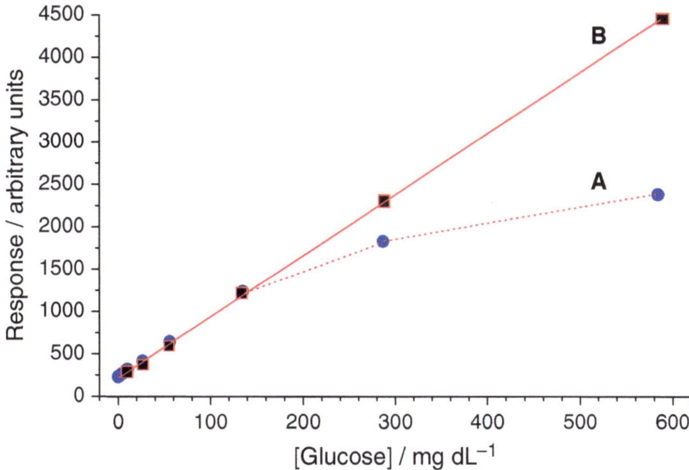

Fig. 2.24 Response-concentration profiles for different glucosensors where oxygen represents (**a**) or does not represent (**b**) a limiting reagent

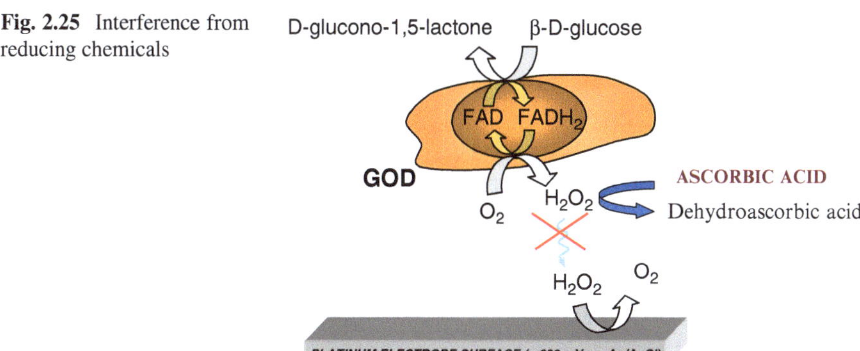

Fig. 2.25 Interference from reducing chemicals

Extremes in pH

Each enzyme exhibits optimal activity within a narrow range of pH. Since the redox processes in both GOD and GDH are pH-dependent (H^+ ions are involved in the reactions), low or high pH values may alter the kinetics with which glucose is oxidised on the test strip. Extreme deviations from the pH of a normal blood sample (7.35–7.45) can, therefore, affect the output of blood glucose meters.

The reagent mix that is dispensed onto the sensor surface contains buffering agents that are typically sufficient to maintain the pH within the range required for optimal enzyme activity. As shown by Tang et al. for a number of systems currently on the market [25], the buffer capacity of the test strip normally allows accurate measurements even with bloods whose pH is as low as 6.97 or as high as 7.84.

However, potential risk still exists in critically ill patients with severe acidosis or other acid–base disorders. In particular, in diabetic patients with severe ketoacidosis and increased haematocrit due to dehydration, the combined effects of pH and haematocrit may result in misleading glucose readings.

A lack of pH interference with glucose measurements may reflect the use of adequate buffering agents, mediators whose redox chemistry is pH-independent (e.g. ferricyanide), enzymes with high activity within a broader range of pH, or other factors in the test-strip biochemistry or physical design.

Interferents Acting at the Redox Mediator Level

The chemical stability of the mediator is an essential requirement for manufacturing highly accurate and precise test strips. However, under certain circumstances a number of undesired processes independent of glucose concentration have the potential to alter the redox state of the mediator. An overview of the most significant interferents acting at the mediator level is reported in what follows.

Humidity

The performances of a blood glucose sensor can be heavily affected by humidity whenever its absorption into the reaction chamber of the strip generates favourable conditions for a glucose-independent reduction of the mediator:

$$\left[\mathrm{Fe^{III}(CN)_6}\right]^{3-} \underset{\text{generic reducing compound}}{\overset{\text{Humid environment+}}{\longrightarrow}} \left[\mathrm{Fe^{II}(CN)_6}\right]^{4-}$$

This is readily reflected in a non-specific current term that adds to the glucose-specific one (Fig. 2.26) and that, consequently, leads to an overestimation of the glycaemic levels.

As an example of the interfering action of humidity, one may cite the case of the first generation of GlucoMen LX and GLUCOFIX sensors, where the ferricyanide mediator is deposited on a gold working electrode and used in combination with the GOD enzyme. To minimise the background current, the mediator salt is dispensed onto the test strip surface in its fully oxidised form (i.e. $[\mathrm{Fe^{III}(CN)_6}]^{3-}$). In dry conditions (i.e. until the strips are kept in their own—desiccant-containing—vials), the iron nucleus of the complex is stable in such a +3 oxidation state. However, as these products are improperly manipulated and the vial cap left open for several hours in a humid environment, the moisture drives the foregoing processes, which dramatically deteriorate the accuracy of the measurements. Currently, the resistance of the strips against exposure to a humid environment has been strongly improved through a minor modification implemented in the dispensed chemistry.

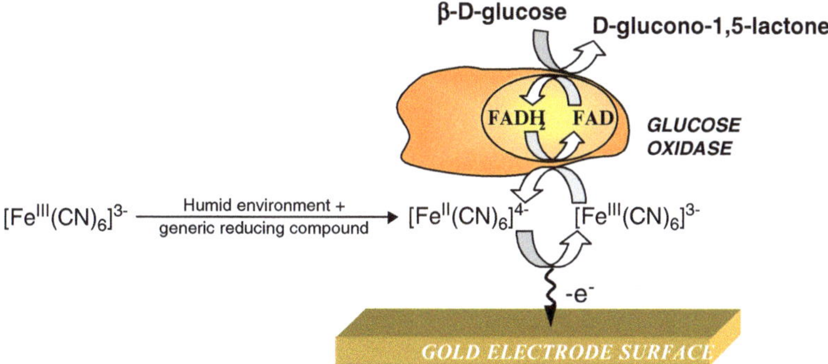

Fig. 2.26 Mechanism explaining overestimation of blood glucose concentrations in sensors exposed to high humidity levels

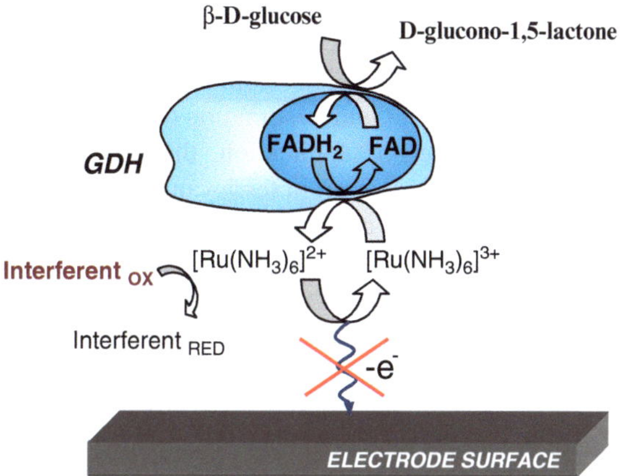

Fig. 2.27 "Consumption" of reduced form of mediator by oxidising chemical

Generic Oxidising Compounds

Often, molecules that exhibit an intrinsic electrochemical activity are regarded as possible interferents only because they are susceptible to direct oxidation (or reduction) at the electrode surface. Nevertheless, one should bear in mind that the interfering mechanism can also be different. The use of mediators with a low formal potential can be extremely useful to minimise the direct electro-oxidation/reduction of endogenous or exogenous chemicals. The problem with these redox reagents is that one such chemical might be sufficiently oxidising to directly react with the reduced form of the mediator. In other words, the interferent might compete with the working electrode for re-oxidising the mediator. In a sensor where GDH is combined with a low formal potential mediator [such as ruthenium (III) hexaammine or a quinone] (Fig. 2.27), this kind of interference would directly come from the oxygen dissolved in the blood sample. The crucial aspect is that the potential at which the working electrode would be polarised is not sufficiently high

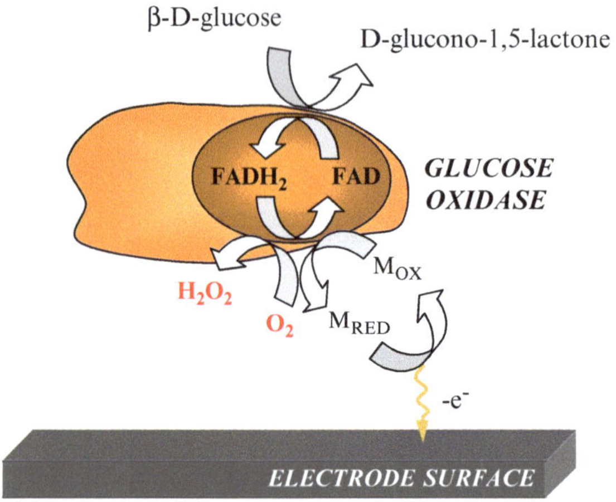

Fig. 2.28 Competition between redox mediator and molecular oxygen for re-oxidation of $FADH_2$ in GOD-mediated glucosensors

to re-oxidise the reduced interferent back to its original form. The fraction of the electrons originally 'stolen' from the glucose would therefore be irreparably lost, with the consequent underestimation of blood sugar levels.

In its first sensor application, the FAD-GDH from *A. terreus* was used in combination with potassium ferricyanide specifically because the oxidation state of this mediator is not affected by oxygen over the time scale of the measurements [10]. Other mediators, such as hexaammine ruthenium(III) or various quinones, were excluded because of their susceptibility to direct re-oxidation by dissolved O_2.

The optimal redox potential of the mediator should be in the range $-0.2\ V < E°' < +0.1\ V$ (versus Ag/AgCl) [11]. Note that several commercially available strips use non-conventional reference electrodes but pseudo-reference ones (inert conductor counter/reference electrodes; see section "Counter/Reference Electrodes"). The potential actually applied at the working electrode surface might therefore significantly differ from the values in the range stated previously.

Oxygen (GOD-Based Glucosensors Only)

Besides the mechanism described previously, oxygen can also interfere with the redox mediator according to a different path. By definition, so-called fast mediators such as ferricyanide are capable of exchanging electrons with the enzyme cofactor more rapidly than O_2, the natural cosubstrate of GOD. However, a certain competition from dissolved oxygen for re-oxidising the reduced form of the cofactor ($FADH_2$) must always be taken into account (Fig. 2.28). Interestingly, the strips are optimised to perform best when the blood sample is the capillary one, and its oxygen partial pressure (pO_2) lays within the characteristic range of 60–90 mmHg. On one hand, when the pO_2 in the blood sample is particularly low, oxygen competes with the mediator less than expected. In such cases, the strips tend to overestimate the blood sugar level. On the other hand, when the pO_2 is particularly high ($>>$ 100 mmHg, e.g. for O_2 -saturated blood samples), oxygen competes with the redox mediator much more than expected. As previously discussed, the potential at which the working electrode is polarised would not be sufficiently high to oxidise the H_2O_2 back to molecular oxygen, with the resulting underestimation of blood glucose levels.

From the mechanism described earlier, it becomes clear how important it is to perform quality control tests on strips using tonometered blood samples (i.e. normally within the range 70–90 mmHg).

Interestingly, FAD-GDH systems are unaffected by pO_2 since O_2 is not able to re-oxidise the reduced form of FAD, when this cofactor is embedded into the active site of GDH [10].

Interferents Acting at Electrode Surface Level

Electrochemical Interferents

Here, the definition of electrochemical interferent applies to those endogenous or exogenous chemicals in blood that, instead of non-specifically reacting with either an enzyme or redox mediator, disturb the measurement of blood glucose concentrations by directly acting at the electrode level. This class of interferents comprises not only molecules that exhibit an intrinsic electrochemical activity in the low potential region (where most of the mediators work) but also electro-inactive species such as cholesterol and triglycerides.

Electrochemically active chemicals can cause false high glucose readings by donating non-glucose-derived electrons to the sensor. At very high concentrations, lipids strongly affect the accuracy of the measurements for two specific reasons: first, they represent a significant percentage of liquid sample that enters the capillary chamber of the sensor (i.e. less glucose molecules can reach the electrode); second, being adsorbed at the electrode surface, they can interfere with all electron transfer processes.

Of the compounds listed in Table 2.8, those most likely to electrochemically interfere are ascorbate, acetaminophen and urate. Strips using a carbon working electrode poised at potentials between -0.1 and $+0.2$ V versus Ag/AgCl, with fast mediators having redox potentials between -0.2 and $+0.1$ V versus Ag/AgCl, do not oxidise urate or acetaminophen; however, virtually all commercial strips cross-react with ascorbate.

One possible way to minimise the adverse effects of these interferents is to introduce into the test strip a secondary working electrode, largely identical to the main one (in terms of electrodic material, mediator, buffering agents, etc.) but lacking the glucose-reacting enzyme. While the current recorded at the primary electrode depends on both glucose-specific and non-specific process, the current measured at the ‘blank’ electrode only accounts for processes that are independent of glucose concentration. The differential current is, therefore, free of this kind of interference. This strategy is adopted, for example, by the StatStrip platform from Nova Biomedical.

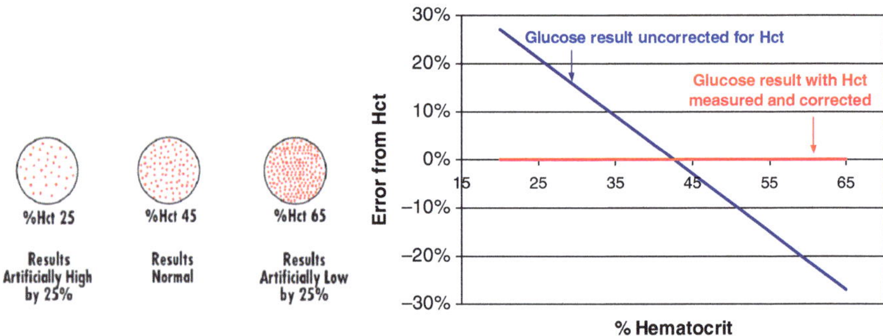

Fig. 2.29 Influence of haematocrit on response of blood glucose strips

Haematocrit Dependence

Haematocrit (the percentage of blood volume occupied by erythrocytes) has a marked effect on the outcome of the strip-based assay for a number of reasons. When GOD is the enzyme of choice, oxygen from erythrocytes can compete with the redox mediator for re-oxidising the enzyme cofactor. Moreover, because of the higher viscosity of bloods containing high levels of haematocrit, the diffusion of all reacting species at the strip surface is slowed down. Finally, because of its corpuscular nature, haematocrit physically limits access to the electrode surface and thus changes the portion of the working electrode surface that is active for transducing the enzyme/glucose reaction.

The allowable haematocrit range for electrochemical blood glucose test strips varies with the strip design. Systems with no haematocrit correction feature typically work properly provided that the haematocrit is in the 25–55% range. In contrast, the most sophisticated meters can now minimise the haematocrit dependence of their response. By means of interelectrode impedance measurements, the actual haematocrit level is evaluated and then used to compensate the final blood sugar outcome. For this reason, these glucose meters can operate on bloods whose haematocrit ranges between 0% and 70%. Both unusually low and unusually high haematocrit levels compromise the accuracy of blood glucose quantitation, as schematically depicted in Fig. 2.29.

Practical Aspects in Glucose Sensor Design

Most commercial blood glucose sensors are based on tiny electrochemical cells that require small sample volumes (0.3–4.0 μL), utilise capillary fill and comprise a stabilised enzyme/redox mediator mix. The strips fill reproducibly with blood in less than 3 s (typically in less than 1 s) and generate results in 5–30 s (accuracy 5–10% versus a laboratory standard). They also provide a plethora of additional features, including the following:

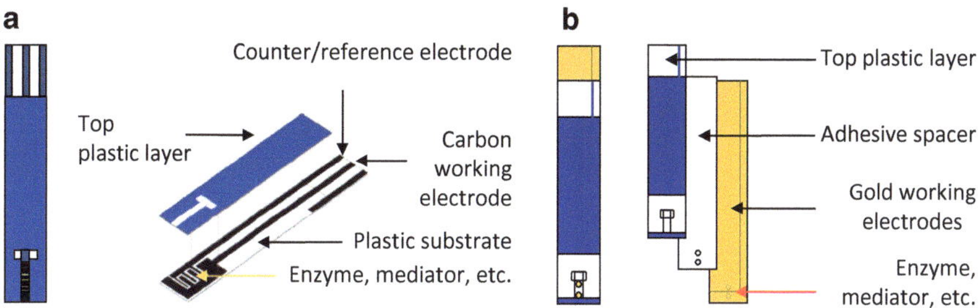

Fig. 2.30 Layer-by-layer structure of different glucose test strips: (**a**) GlucoMen sensor; (**b**) GLUCOFIX sensor

(a) Automatic (non-visual) fill detection;
(b) Code-free operation;
(c) The option to fill the strip with at least two blood aliquots;
(d) On-strip haematocrit compensation.

The following sections describe practical aspects involved in the design of test strips (mainly from Ref. [11]). The working area of the strip is made by patterning the sensing elements onto a plastic substrate material (Fig. 2.30).

At least a working electrode and a counter/reference electrode can be found, either adjacent to each other or separate on facing plastic substrates. An independent counter electrode and an additional (baseline) working electrode may also be included in the electrochemical cell. A small-volume capillary chamber ($< 1\ \mu L$) is formed over the plastic substrate(s) and the electrodes, often by means of a spacer such as a pressure-sensitive adhesive and a cover layer. The strip chemistry, consisting of an enzyme, a redox mediator and other components, is distributed (in dry form) within the capillary chamber and generally covers at least the working electrode. Some of the strips include fill detection electrodes, which are vestigial electrodes enabling the meter to detect that the strip is sufficiently filled with blood to initiate the assay.

Plastic Substrates

The strip body is generally constructed of a thin piece of plastic. It serves as a foundation for the electrodes, which are generally deposited by either screen-printing or vapour deposition. The substrate material has a high glass transition temperature, so that high-temperature process steps (e.g. drying after application of strip reagents in liquid form) do not cause distortion of the plastic or its electrodes. Its mechanical strength allows physical handling (e.g. insertion into the glucose meter) yet provides for machinability, such that small sections can be rapidly and accurately cut from a large sheet of material during strip production. The most widely used materials are polyesters.

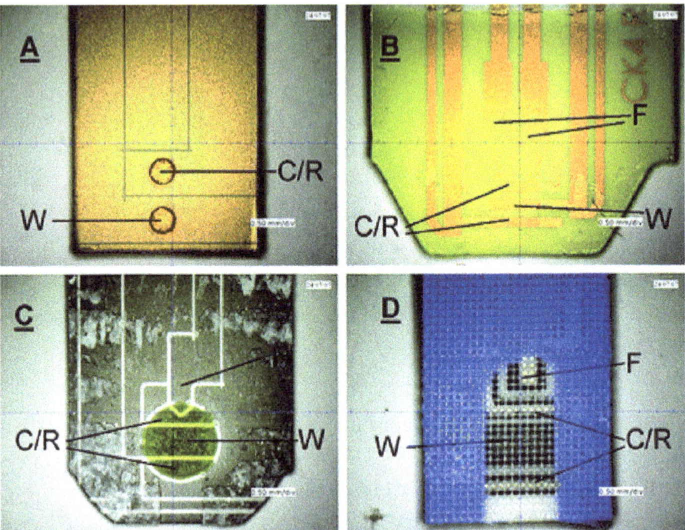

Fig. 2.31 Small-volume electrochemically blood glucose monitoring strips with their *top cover* layer removed. *W*, *C/R* and *F* indicate working, counter/reference and fill detection electrodes, respectively

Working Electrodes

The working electrode is most commonly obtained by screen-printing a carbon-based ink (i.e. a mixture of carbon particles and a polyester binder) or by vapour deposition of gold (Au) or palladium (Pd). Common electrode configurations are illustrated in Fig. 2.31.

The working electrode area must be known and constant for the strips to be reproducibly sensitive to glucose. This area is generally defined by the electrode deposition process (i.e. a reproducible area is deposited or scribed), by an insulating dielectric overlayer that masks a reproducible fraction of the working electrode, or by a combination of the two. By means of the most advanced thin-film technologies extremely small sensing elements can be reproducibly fabricated. These, combined with the tiny volume of the capillary μ-chamber, allow the blood glucose concentration to be assayed employing sample volumes as small as 0.3 μL, a quantity that can be painlessly obtained by the patient. Generally, the active reagents are deposited over the working electrode, but sometimes they are admixed into the conducting materials. The distance between working and counter/reference electrode is minimised, both to reduce the sample volume and the interelectrode electrolytic resistance.

Counter/Reference Electrodes

The commercially available electrochemical strips usually comprise two electrode devices; the counter and reference electrode functions are combined in a single electrode. The counter/reference electrode can be coplanar with the working electrode (in which case it often lies upstream of the working electrode) or it can be located on an opposite wall of the capillary cell, such that it faces the working electrode. Most commonly, these counter/reference electrodes are obtained using either a silver/silver chloride (Ag/AgCl) or an inert conductor.

Ag/AgCl counter/reference electrodes are formed by screen-printing an Ag/AgCl ink, which consists of a mixture of Ag and AgCl particles in a polyester binding material. Here glucose-derived electrons react with AgCl to produce Ag, thereby ejecting chloride ions into the sample chamber. Such electrodes are generally designed to have an available Coulombic capacity of reducible AgCl that exceeds by approximately 1 order of magnitude the greatest charge the strip will pass in an actual glucose assay.

The inert conductor counter/reference electrodes are generally made of the material of the working electrode of a particular strip, such as screen-printed carbon or vapour-deposited Au or Pd. This reduces costs because the working and counter/reference electrodes are deposited in the same manufacturing step. The counter/reference electrode functions by reducing part of the excess oxidised mediator in which it is bathed. Thus, initially, in the dry state, both the working and the counter/reference electrodes are coated with a large excess of oxidised mediator. When glucose-containing blood fills the strip, a small fraction of the excess mediator is reduced via the enzyme-catalysed reaction with glucose. The working electrode oxidises the reduced mediator while the counter/reference reduces part of the oxidised mediator from the large available pool. Thus, inert conductor counter/reference electrodes are feasible only in the presence of a large stoichiometric excess of the oxidised mediator over the glucose.

Thick-Film Versus Thin-Film Sensor Production Technology

If compared to thick-film (screen-printing) technologies, thin-film deposition processes are characterised by a much higher resolution, which makes it possible to obtain smaller yet perfectly defined and extremely reproducible sensors.

In screen-printing, similar levels of resolution can only be obtained by combining the so-called classical screen-printing methodology for massively producing the sensors with a subsequent laser ablation step that provides the final electrodes' interdistance and surface size.

The sensors produced using high-resolution techniques possess a number of advantageous features.

First, the resulting glucosensors are so reproducible and accurate that the end-user is not requested to perform manual calibrations. This clearly simplifies the measuring protocol while also preventing unskilled patients from committing errors.

Second, the possibility of producing smaller electrodes without compromising the general analytical performance of the test offers the possibility of detecting glucose in sub-microlitre volume samples. This directly translates into a need for smaller lancets, which reduces the pain and the discomfort associated with finger pricking.

Third, due to the smaller size of the glucose-responding electrode, a strip of classical dimensions can integrate multiple sensing electrodes, thereby enabling multi-analyte detection or effective correction of interferences associated with either electrochemically active species or haematocrit.

Reagents

Reagents are commonly dispensed by an ink-jet printing technology over at least the working electrode, but they may cover the entire capillary chamber. In some strips (e.g. Precision Xtra) the reagents are mixed directly with the conducting carbon ink and the mixture is co-deposited onto the strip. Reagents include at least an enzyme and often a mediator for oxidising glucose; they might also include surfactants to minimise the strip-filling time, enzyme stabilisers and film-forming agents, among others. Typical surface-active agents enhancing strip-filling include surfactants such as Triton X-100. Enzyme stabilisers may include compounds such as monosodium glutamate, trehalose, bovine serum albumin, and buffering agents that maintain the enzyme at a favourable pH during storage. Film-forming agents such as silica are reputed to improve haematocrit performance.

Calibration

Strips are factory-calibrated as follows. Blood samples at low, medium and high glucose concentrations are analysed using both the blood glucose test strips and a reference method. The strip response (electrical current or charge) is then plotted versus the glucose reference value. The resulting slope and intercept are finally used to select a strip code for use in the meter or to accept or reject the strip lot for codeless systems.

Commercially available strips are required to meet the accuracy and precision criteria dictated by the ISO protocol 15197 [79]. They must perform precisely and accurately over the entire range of clinical interest (i.e. 20–600 mg/dL or 1–33 mM), typically displaying coefficients of variation (CV) of 2–5% for replicate measurements. The CV is generally higher at very low glucose concentrations, where strip background (signal in the absence of glucose) represents a significant and variable contribution.

Alternate Site Testing

The ability to accurately detect capillary blood glucose from an alternative site (e.g. palm or forearm) is of great value for those people who are unable to obtain capillary finger-prick blood samples or those who want to experience less discomfort (pain) while monitoring their diabetes. The pain associated with skin lancing at alternative sites is smaller due to the lower enervation of these areas:

Fingers: highly enervated (pain issues)
Forearm: 20–25% of finger nerve levels
Palm: 75% of finger nerve density

One must, however, consider that a time-lag does exist between venous glucose levels and those at non-finger sites. Therefore, sampling from alternative sites is not recommended when glycaemic levels are expected to change rapidly, e.g. after a meal, after taking insulin, or during or after exercise.

Additional Factors Affecting the Quantitation of Blood Glucose Levels

Some important sources of error in the quantitation of blood glucose levels were discussed earlier, including dependence of the signal on haematocrit and on electrochemical interferences. Other sources of error include signal dependence on the temperature, skin contamination with glucose or other sugars, use of improper devices or measuring protocols, and imperfect application of the blood samples.

Haemolysis

The term haemolysis indicates the premature breakdown of RBCs caused, for example, by the excessive milking or squeezing of the fingertip after lancing of the site. Haemolysis of a specimen can result in the collection of tissue fluids along with the blood. The consequent dilution of the sample adversely affects the test results (underestimation of blood glucose concentration). Haemolysis can also be induced by specific pathologies, including autoimmune haemolytic anaemia (due to drugs or incompatibility between blood groups), trauma associated with mechanical aortic valve prostheses, abnormalities in the membrane of the red blood cells, and hypersplenism.

Temperature

Both the enzyme reactivity and the intrinsic electrochemistry of all (bio)chemical reagents are temperature-dependent. Possible signal variations associated with temperature changes are, therefore, compensated by measuring the temperature during the assay and applying a correction algorithm. Coulometric systems have an intrinsically lower temperature dependence compared to amperometric ones. The temperature compensation in amperometric systems is, however, quite accurate and makes negligible any difference in the operating temperature ranges (typically approximately 5–40°C).

Skin Contamination

Skin surface contamination is a significant problem because a blood droplet can dissolve the glucose left on the fingertips by foods in which the concentration of glucose is particularly high (e.g. grapes). The skin-contamination problem has been amplified by the trend of using smaller blood sample sizes, which leads to increased solute/solvent ratios. Users should always wash their hands with soapy water and then carefully dry the skin prior to lancing.

Peritoneal Dialysis

Peritoneal dialysis involves injection into the peritoneum of an iso-osmotic fluid rich in icodextrin, a polymer of maltose. This leads to a significant elevation of the blood levels of non-glucose sugar. Strips made using the GDH/PQQ enzyme-cofactor pair are known to heavily cross-react with maltose and, therefore, must not be used by diabetic patients on peritoneal dialysis.

Miscoding

Miscoding occurs when the calibration code (assigned to the strip vial during production) is incorrectly entered into the meter. This is addressed by automatic coding chips supplied with the strip vial; however, miscoding is still possible if a coding chip is not used. The best solution is in either no-coding or autocoding strips. On one hand, no-coding strips rely on a rigorous selection process during production that limits sensitivity variations; on the other hand, autocoding strips carry a readable mark that allows the meter to automatically assign the code to each lot of strips.

Strip Filling

To obtain reliable results, it is of crucial importance for the strip to be completely filled with blood when the electrochemical assay commences. This is obvious for coulometric strips, which rely upon a precisely known sample volume to calculate a glucose concentration. It is equally true for amperometric strips, where partial working electrode coverage by blood will introduce an error (underestimation). Formerly, filling was visually confirmed by the user; today, it is automated to reduce the likelihood of user error and to make the assay faster. Fill detection is realised in electrochemical strips by the following methods:

(I) Positioning the counter/reference electrode downstream (in the sample flow path) from the working electrode. This condition guarantees that the working electrode will be completely covered with blood before the electrochemical circuit is completed by exposure of the counter/reference electrode to the blood.

(II) Using identical dual working electrodes, one downstream from the other in the sample flow path. The signal from the two electrodes can then be compared and the measurement rejected if not sufficiently similar.

(III) Adding another sensing electrode downstream from the working electrode. When current is detected at the sensing electrode, the strip is deemed full.

Reference Methods

YSI Glucose Analysers

The YSI glucose analysers (introduced by Yellow Spring Instruments, Yellow Springs, OH, in 1974) served historically as and still represent the gold standard with which the accuracy of other glucose analysers are compared (Fig. 2.32).

The core of YSI glucose analysers is their glucose monitoring probe, which consists of layered polymeric membranes (one of which is GOD-modified) covering a Pt wire electrode (where H_2O_2 is electro-oxidised to O_2, Fig. 2.33).

The membrane contacting the analysed solution, which is 30 times diluted when blood or serum is analysed, is made of polycarbonate. Other than preventing fouling, this membrane reduces the glucose influx, thereby extending the dynamic range and the useful life of the probe. The GOD, which catalyses the glucose conversion and generates H_2O_2, is immobilised on the Pt side of this outer polycarbonate membrane. The inner membrane is made of cellulose acetate. It excludes most interferents but, being permeable to H_2O_2, allows its diffusion to the Pt electrode.

YSI glucose analysers introduced two significant design principles that were adopted in later flow analysers and in implantable glucose electrodes. First, the influx of glucose is reduced by dilution of the analysed solution and by the

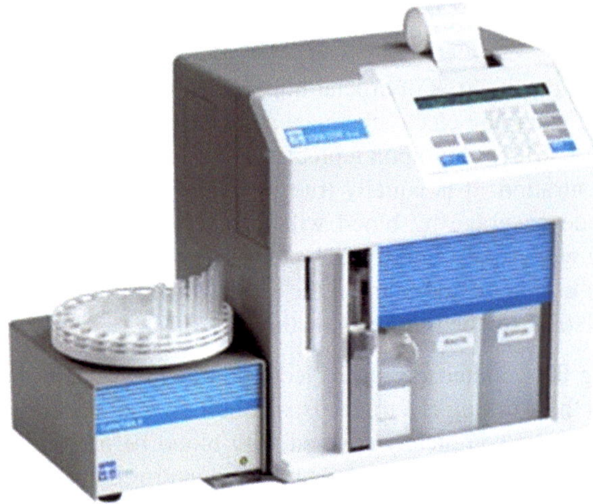

Fig. 2.32 YSI 2300 STAT Plus glucose and lactate analyzer

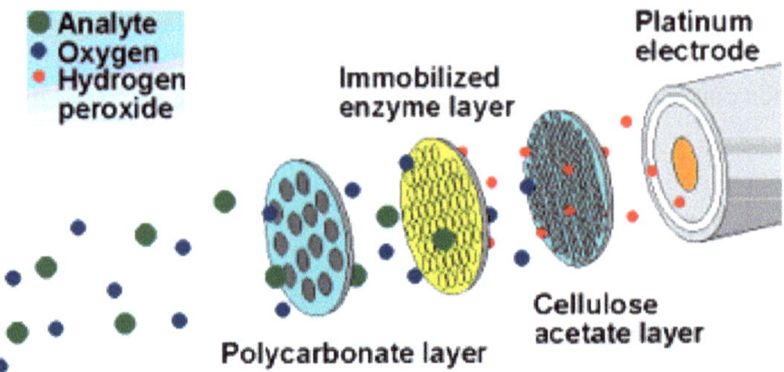

Fig. 2.33 Layer-by-layer structure of YSI glucose monitoring probe

outer polycarbonate membrane sufficiently for all of the glucose passing the outer membrane to react with dissolved O_2. This is achieved even though the saturating concentration of O_2 in water at 25°C is approximately only 0.2 mM, while the glucose concentration in the undiluted blood of a diabetic patient can be as high as 30 mM (i.e. 150 times higher). The second important principle introduced by YSI analysers concerns the amount of GOD to be bound (via glutaraldehyde cross-linking) onto the enzymatic membrane. Immobilisation of an initially large excess of GOD ensures complete conversion of the glucose that passes the outer membrane, even after most of the initial GOD activity is lost.

The current YSI 2300 STAT glucose analyser utilises a 25 μL sample, has a throughput of one sample per 100 s and measures glucose concentrations up to 50 mM, with an error lower than ± 2% or 0.2 mM. The working life of its membrane is 21 days.

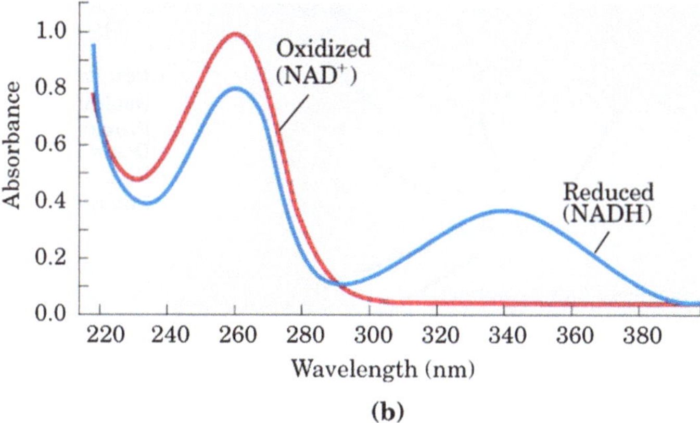

Fig. 2.34 Absorption spectra of NAD^+ and NADH

Hexokinase Method

The hexokinase method is another reference method for the determination of glucose concentration. This method relies on the combined use of two enzymes, hexokinase and glucose-6-phosphate dehydrogenase, which ensures a high specificity toward D-glucose. The working principle is schematically represented below:

$$\text{Glucose} + \text{ATP} \overset{\text{Hexokinase}}{\rightarrow} \text{Glucose-6-phosphate} + \text{ADP}$$

$$\text{Glucose-6-phosphate} + \text{NAD}^+ \underset{\text{dehydrogenase}}{\overset{\text{Glucose-6-phosphate}}{\rightarrow}} \text{6-Phosphogluconate} + \text{NADH} + \text{H}^+$$

In the presence of adenosine triphosphate (ATP), the hexokinase catalyses the phosphorylation of D-glucose. The resulting glucose-6-phosphate is then further processed by glucose-6-phosphate dehydrogenase in the presence of NAD^+, with the production of 6-phosphogluconate and NADH. The concentration of NADH, which is directly proportional to the blood sugar level, is finally quantified spectrophotometrically at 340 nm (Fig. 2.34).

Besides glucose, fructose and mannose can also react in primary reaction. However, glucose-6-phosphate dehydrogenase is specific exclusively to glucose-6-phosphate; thus, phosphorylated fructose and mannose do not react in indicator reaction.

Hospital Glucose Monitoring Systems

Recently a new class of glucose meters, specifically designed to deal with aggressive environments such as hospital wards treating in-patients on multiple medications, has been made commercially available by the most important industry players.

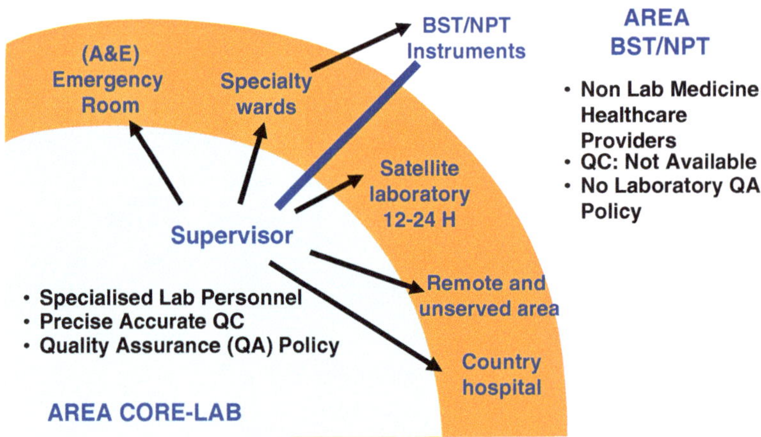

Fig. 2.35 Achieving the highest level of quality of process through connectivity

They belong to a new segment of diagnostic devices known as point-of-care testing (POCT), that encompasses all testing conducted at or near the site of the patient by healthcare professionals (HCPs) in many different hospital and community settings.

The POCT philosophy relies on the assumption that faster results lead to faster decisions making and, finally, to better patient outcomes. To successfully accomplish such objectives, it is believed that POCT analysers must fulfil the quality criteria of conventional analysers in terms of performance. Moreover, they should be user-friendly and easy to maintain, even by non-specialised personnel; as such, the technology used in POCT is designed to minimise the need for technical skills and overall turnaround time (TAT) compared with the equipment in use in the central laboratory.

A key factor to achieve the requirements mentioned above, aside from the superior analytical quality of the employed biosensors, is the supervision of the overall workflow, which consists of (1) an analytical phase, (2) the quality control (QC) status of the test, (3) the traceability of relevant control material, (4) identification of the operators and clinical validation of tests by the central laboratory staff (Fig. 2.35).

It is also crucial to guarantee accessibility to electronic medical records (EMRs) for both downloading and uploading information such as patient admission, transfer and discharge and, obviously, test results. Effective implementation of such a level of coordination requires both connectivity capabilities on board of the POCT device or meter and the data management solutions able to communicate bidirectionally between the device and the data management system [26]. To date, point-of-care diagnostic vendors and partners have faced this integration problem individually and have conceived unique solutions. Any healthcare institution embarking on incorporating multivendor point-of-care diagnostic devices into their diagnostic testing facilities has had to face the equipment and management costs of multiple integrated solutions, and this issue has created a significant barrier to the broad adoption of POCT in diverse clinical scenarios. In February 2009, 49 healthcare institutions, point-of-care diagnostic vendors, in vitro diagnostic (IVD) system vendors and system integrators established the Connectivity Industry Consortium (CIC) to resolve this POCT diagnostic integration problem. The result was a set of seamless so-called plug-and-play communication standards that are becoming the foundation for POCT connectivity across the healthcare continuum.

Nowadays, to achieve a high level of integration and interoperability among multivendor IVD applications, compliance with the international standards described in the CLSI/CIC document POCT1-2A, recently approved by the International Federation of Clinical Chemistry and Laboratory Medicine (IFCC) is highly recommended. POCT1-2A requirements include, among others, the use of HL7, a de facto messaging standard that enables disparate healthcare applications to exchange key sets of clinical and administrative data. HL7, a protocol working on the seventh layer (application layer) of the ISO/OSI model of communication, allows seamless multivendor interoperability and therefore provides healthcare institutions with a degree of mastery over data and coordination. The latter is a must for harmonising care and sharing information about diagnosis and treatments between separate institutions. Such a scenario, often referred to as continuity of care, is a prerequisite for delivery of efficient individualised medicine that will largely benefit from a strong multidisciplinary and interdepartmental team approach to patient care according to the best clinical practices recommended by new, evidence based medicine guidelines or directives.

The College of American Pathologists (CAP) produced an instrument survey in April 2007 detailing features of available POCT glucose devices for hospital applications, desired meter specifications to bridge the gap with an ideal product concept and, finally, comments from manufacturers. The manufacturers of the bedside glucose testing systems featured in CAP's survey have responded to the current demands with new instruments and features, from multiple measuring wells to wireless capabilities.

For example, Nova Biomedical recently introduced a hospital handheld glucose meter that fulfils the aforementioned requirements. The device, commercially known as StatStrip, is a system used to address the need for improved test accuracy and freedom from interference, a requirement made crucial by the increased use of tight glycaemic control protocols (TGC) in critical care medicine (Fig. 2.36). In fact, the use of handheld POCT glucose devices for monitoring patient glucose levels in critically ill patients on intravenous insulin allows for rapid clinical decision making and immediate treatment responses. However, target glucose concentrations are often tighter for this patient population compared to self-testing diabetic patients using handheld meters to dose subcutaneous insulin. As a result greater meter accuracy is required in order to avoid insulin-dosing errors. In addition, patients in the ICU are on multiple medications, often have abnormal haematocrit, and are ventilated, all of which may affect the performance of handheld glucose

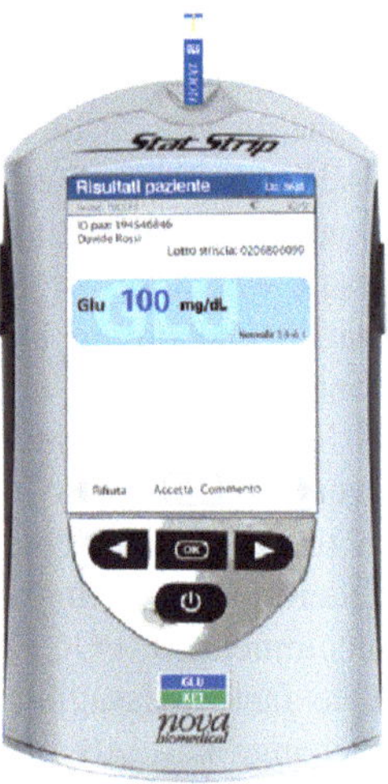

Fig. 2.36 The StatStrip glucose and Ketone monitoring system

meters. Oxygen tension and pH may affect a limited number of glucose meter technologies [67, 68]. Several studies have confirmed that interfering substances such as medications used in the critical care setting or abnormal patient haematocrit levels can adversely affect the performance of almost all glucose meter technologies available [69–71]. Low haematocrit levels can give rise to falsely elevated glucose readings and conversely high haematocrit levels can give rise to falsely low glucose readings. It is well known that some of the enzymes used in glucose meters are not specific for glucose and can give falsely elevated results when other non-glucose sugars are present in patient samples. It is also increasingly recognized that a wide range of endogenous and exogenous substances present in the blood of critically ill patients can donate electrons which initiate the electrochemical reaction and cause interference with glucose results, giving elevated values.

There is an increased risk of dosing errors occurring if the mean %bias of glucose meter readings differ by >15 % from the true value [72]. A recent study has indicated that many commonly used meters exceed this bias in a critical care population [73]. Therefore the use of meters affected by haematocrit and non-glucose or electrochemical interferences may result in errors in patient care and contribute to an increased risk of undetected hypoglycaemia. In critical care, patients are often sedated, and hypoglycaemia may not be obvious and clinical signs may be difficult or impossible to recognise. Consequences of hypoglycaemia include cognitive dysfunction, seizures and death [74]. The poor accuracy of commonly used glucose meters in a critical care setting has been the subject of regulatory concern and a recent statement by Emergency Care Research Institute (ECRI) in association with the FDA state that users should evaluate the performance of blood glucose meters prior to selection for use with critically ill patients. In February 2013 CLSI published new guidelines CPOCT 12 A3 outlining the approach to take for the evaluation of POC glucose meters for use in acute and chronic care facilities [75]. Nova

Biomedical's new handheld POC StatStrip system, specifically designed for use in a hospitalised setting, has been reported to give good accuracy in analytical studies and has been shown to be unaffected by hematocrit and other interfering substances [76–78]. The design of the technology of this meter incorporates a glucose specific reaction zone and two additional separate reaction zones, which measure and correct for hematocrit and other interfering substances such as maltose, galactose, acetaminophen, ascorbic acids and uric acid. Glucose readings are corrected against the readings from the interference zones eliminating the influence of hematocrit and chemical interference on clinical accuracy. The StatStrip features a 6-s measuring time, 1.2 mL sample volume, highlights abnormal and critical results, and requires no calibration coding. In addition, the system eliminates errors due to overdosing or undersampling. Besides glucose, the Nova's device can also measure the blood concentration of ketone bodies by quantifying beta-hydroxybutirate. Ketone bodies are produced by fatty acid metabolism in hepatic mitochondria during a range of physiological and pathological conditions. Monitoring ketones in DKA (Diabetes Keto-Acidosis) and critically ill patients can aid patient management and a POCT device could aid rapid targeted clinical decision making provided good quality results are obtained. Analytical studies performed according to CLSI guidelines (EP5, EP17, EP9 and EP7) have demonstrated that the StatStrip meter provides fast and easy blood ketone monitoring from capillary samples whilst guaranteeing good analytical performances [65].

The recent business partnership with A.Menarini Diagnostics (AMD), has provided an opportunity for AMD to distribute the StatStrip hospital meter in several European countries. This has provided an opportunity for AMD to deliver a "complete POCT diagnostic solution" comprising the StatStrip system, which addresses the analytical and clinical quality issues, and the NetCare 2.0 IT platform, which effectively addresses the need for high quality patient information and data processing. The fusion of the two products into a unique commercial package, enables a total-quality approach in the delivery of decentralised diagnostics by improving the remote control of both StatStrip and other third-party POCT instruments, carried out by central laboratory staff (Fig. 2.37). More specifically, NetCare 2.0 guarantees an electronic support for inventory, quality control, training and administrative responsibility and provides extensive device management and data reporting functions. In addition, it provides easy access to audit data for regulatory compliance.

NetCare 2.0 fulfils clinical governance and many national guidelines for POCT and enables a link to LIS/HIS IT platforms in order to allow for the secure transmission of results to EMRs.

State-of-the-art, alternative solutions from other market players include the Accu-check Inform II (meter) and Cobas IT 1,000 (data management) Roche Diagnostics combo solution and the Precision PCX meter and the PrecisionWeb data management package supplied by Abbott Diagnostics. In 2004, BST a German company, introduced a unique POCT application, namely the first handheld, relatively low-cost electrochemical glucose analyser (Glukometer 3,000) made with

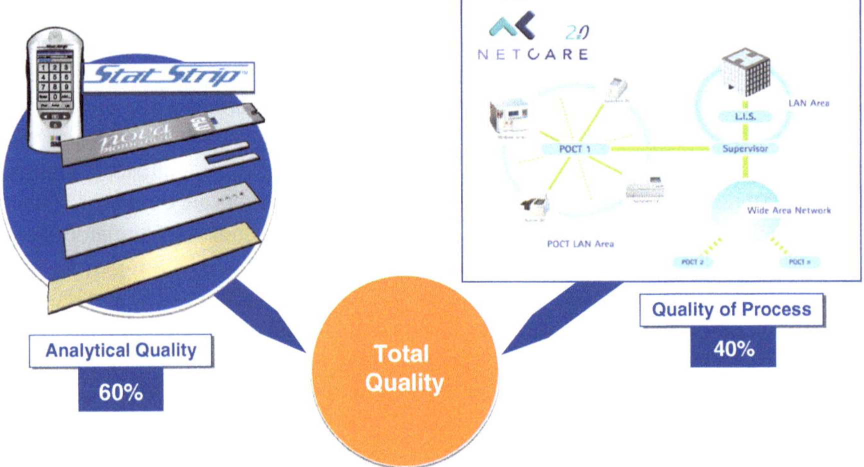

Fig. 2.37 Delivery of total quality at point of need

a biosensor requiring replacement only after 30 days of use or after assays of as many as 1,000 samples. This is made possible by the BTS analyser fluidics, which is designed to initiate cleaning between sampling using a few microlitres of rinsing solution, thereby reducing the biohazardous fluid disposal burden. The heart of the device consists of a unique "multi-way glucose biosensor" that is a combination of a thick film electrode on ceramic with glucose oxidase immobilized onto a special polymer. Glucose oxidase catalyzes glucose oxidation according to the following reaction:

$$\text{Glucose} + 1/2\text{O}_2 \xrightarrow{\text{Glucose oxidase}} \text{Glucono lactone} + \text{H}_2\text{O}_2$$

The GOD enzyme is immobilised in a way that the "disposable biosensor" can measure more than 1,000 samples because of the reversibility of the enzyme metabolism. Each biosensor is delivered and stored dry in a blister packaging at +4 °C and this procedure guarantees a 1 year stability whilst, when the sensor is onboard, the lifetime is 30 days or 1,000 measurements. The replacement of the biosensor is SW-guided and the run-in of a newly placed sensor takes about 60 min. The instrument is calibrated to both capillary and venous blood and the samples to be analysed must be collected through a capillary glass which is afterword placed into a dedicate port. Overall, based upon the results shown in literature [63], it is possible to state that the Glukometer 3,000 can offer a workable compromise between the two different needs of lab-like quality and ability to rapidly test at the point of care at a reasonable price. For such a reason, a precursor of the Glukometer 3000 has been widely employed in East-Germany until 1989 to diagnose all the diabetic patients.

It is worth pointing out that although current technology offers good results in term of sensitivity, dynamic range and detection limits, industry is exploring new technologies based on the nanostructuration of electrochemical sensors to further improve the analytical performances of glucose and other metabolites sensors [84].

Finally, it makes sense to point-out the advent of a new class of devices, specifically designed for the ICU needs, which integrate glucose monitoring with arterial blood gas (ABG) and electrolyte analysis. In fact, periodic measurements of ABG, and electrolytes is a standard of care for patients both in ICU and OR in case of: (1) symptoms of oxygen/carbon dioxide or PH imbalance, (2) prolonged anesthesia, (3) respiratory distress, (4) respiratory, metabolic and kidney diseases, (4) newborns admitted in the NICU with breathing disorders. Small handheld POCT devices available in the market which enable to determine GLU, ABG and electrolytes at the patient's bedside are: (1) the Sphere's Proxima analyser, (2) the Abbott's i-STAT system and (3) the Alere's EPOC.

Gluocose Measurement and Telemedicine

Advocates of healthcare delivered at home, have recently emphasized the need of a policy to enhance the use of home-care, backed by an extensive deployment of ICT (information and communication technologies) infrastructures as a less expensive alternative to hospitalisation. Recent literatures has identified home-base disease management as programmes as an evolving and important part application of telemedicine. In 2008 A.Menarini Diagnostics carried-out a project (C.A.S.E) in co-operation with the Italian National Institute of Health where different devices for measuring blood pressure, heart rate, blood glucose and physical activity where integrated into a single patient unit equipped with a GSM module to periodically transmit the acquired data by using the SMS protocol. The enrolled patients where selected among those discharged from hospital after a major cardiovascular or cerebrovascular event. The system was very well accepted by the patients monitored with a such a system. Another important application where glucose meters are often employed is m-health. M-health is an emerging concept that uses mobile communication devices, tablets, personal digital assistants and other wireless devices. With m-health systems, glucose data can be now automatically collected, transmitted, aggregated with other physiological data and finally presented as actionable information. The reasons why the above mentioned information are not yet widely accepted are reported in the chart below.

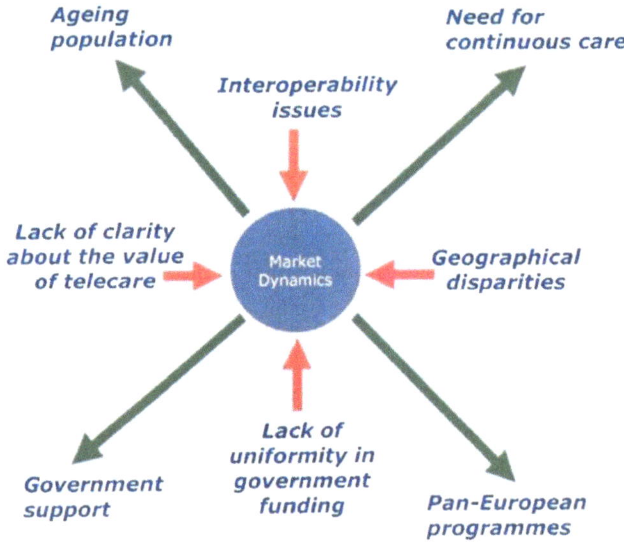

Fig. 2.38

Continuous Glucose Monitoring Systems and Implantable Biosensors

Modern diabetes treatment offer a variety of different therapeutic options and concepts. Moreover, the quality of blood glucose monitors for self-testing has been significantly improved over the past few years. Despite this, there are still diagnostic and therapeutic gaps, in particular for patients treated with insulin, that may have significant effects on the development of acute and/or long-term diabetes complications. More specifically, due to the results of several landmark studies, there is a broad consensus on the importance to devise treatment regimens designed to control glucose excursion targets to achieve and maintain specific glycaemic goals. Notwithstanding this need, the control of diabetes treatment via both HbA1c (a long term marker of metabolic imbalance) and daily blood glucose measurements (SMBG) cannot regularly monitor for glycemic variability and the repeated occurrence of hypoglycaemic episodes and metabolically relevant hyperglycaemic episodes. Systems for continuous glucose monitoring (CGMS), which enable uninterrupted glucose measurements taken at interval of a few minutes (or even less) over several days, can better monitor glycemic variability in order to overcome the diagnostic gap described above and to achieve a stable and predictable metabolic status. Last but not least, CGM, offers an excellent foundation for a dialogue between the physician, diabetes advisor and patient in order to better understand therapeutic effects and behavioural patterns and to recognise insufficiently treated metabolic phases.

Finally, intensive insulin therapy requires several blood glucose measurements per day in order to adjust insulin doses. Even with intensive intermittent monitoring, the number of glucose measurements is limited and some important information can be missed, such as postprandial hyperglycaemia, nocturnal hypoglycaemia and glycaemic variability. A CGMS can act as (1) a glycaemic holter for more adequate insulin adjustment (professional CGMS for personalised therapy), (2) a warning system for better detection of both hypoglycaemic events trends in glucose level (consumer CGMS), (3) an in-line, real-time monitor of blood glucose for critically ill patients (critical CGMS), and ultimately, (4) an automatic closed-loop insulin delivery system (artificial pancreas). It is also very important to distinguish between the diagnostic and therapeutic roles of CGMSs. Earlier devices were not real time, were intended only for occasional use and therefore were only diagnostic. A new generation of inexpensive wireless monitoring systems with real-time display of glucose measurements that address the needs of patients have already been on the market for a decade and may replace SMBG as a therapeutic tool. A typical CGM system consists of the following features:

1. A disposable glucose sensor placed subcutaneously or intravenously, which is worn a few days before replacement;
2. A link from the sensor to a non-implanted transmitter that communicates to a radio receiver;
3. A receiver unit worn like an insulin pump that displays glucose levels on a nearly continuous basis and monitors the rising and falling trends.

The concept of CGM was developed in the mid-1970s with the mobile version of the Biostator, which was basically derived from the Yellow Springs glucose analyser, described in section "CGMS Segmentation", widely employed in biochemistry.

Although it is possible in principle to employ the latest generation of amperometric redox-mediated sensors in any CGM device, the systems presently in use still adopt the first generation of chemistry, namely the method founded on the GOD enzymatic reaction, which converts glucose into gluconic acid with the production of hydrogen peroxidase, which then liberates electrons at the contact of a polarised electrode. The enzyme is immobilised on a polymer matrix that is selective for specific blood substrates and reaction products. The electrode detects an electrical current, which is converted into a glucose concentration. The sensor just described is very interesting in terms of analytical performances because (1) it is able to detect small changes in glucose concentrations and (2) the electrical signal is linear for a wide range of physiological levels.

In general terms it is possible to state that, although the multiple fairly accurate readings of CGM systems are not as accurate as traditional SMBG in point-to-point comparisons, analysis of these multiple readings facilitates retrospective identification of glucose trends throughout the day, and these trends can also be predictive of glucose level in the immediate future. In other words, whereas traditional point-in-time SMBG yields more accurate individual results, CGM data present a more accurate overall assessment of the past, present and immediate future of the glycaemic status [27–29, 44, 50, 56–58].

CGMS Segmentation

A first classification can be made between (1) subcutaneous needle-type sensors and (2) microdialysis-based sensors. In commercially available subcutaneous (needle-type) glucose sensors, the reference electrode is the Ag/AgCl. A typical sensor configuration includes three electrodes: a GOx working electrode, a counter electrode and an AgCl reference electrode. In practise, the previously described thin flexible sensor is inserted directly under the skin. The electro-oxidation of glucose is mediated by either O_2 or an immobilised redox mediator. A glucose flux-limiting membrane overlies at least the working electrode of the sensor. Commercially available solutions are represented by Guardian Real-Time (Medtronic, Minneapolis, Minnesota, US), FreeStyle Navigator (Abbott Diabetes Care) and DexCom STS-7 (DexCom, San Diego, California, US). Microdalysis-based sensors employ a semi-permeable membrane filter (permeable to glucose) in the form of a hollow fibre inserted subcutaneously. An isotonic buffer solution containing no glucose in pumped through the membrane fibre and the glucose in the interstitial fluid (ISF) diffuses through the membrane into the fluid stream by osmotic forces. The glucose concentration in the pumped fluid will approach an equilibrium concentration equal to the glucose concentration in the interstitial fluid. The fluid flowing through the microdialysis membrane is pumped to a glucose-measuring cell. The measuring cell can be exposed to atmospheric oxygen, eliminating the subcutaneous oxygen deficit in a GOx electrochemical sensor using O_2/H_2O_2 as the mediator. It is worth pointing out that one main advantage of this method is that the sensing element is outside the body where biofouling mechanism cannot interfere with the measurement. In any case, to avoid the foreign body reaction due to the insertion of the hollow fibre, a biocompatible microdialysis membrane is a necessity. The lag time introduced by this device can be minimised by maximising the fluid flow rate; however, if the flow is too high, there will not be sufficient time to establish a glucose equilibrium between the pumped fluid and the interstitial fluid. The most important commercially CGM system employing this technology is the GlucoDay and the GlucoMen Day of A.Menarini Diagnostics [62].

From a market perspective, several industry experts have suggested dividing the CGMS space into three major segments: (a) consumer segment, (b) professional segment and (2) critical care segment.

Typically a consumer CGM is based on a catheter-tip measuring technology; the sensor can be attached either on the upper arm or the abdomen and sends interstitial glucose levels to the receiver, which stores and displays glucose data. Trends in glucose level are displayed graphically, whilst audio warnings can be set to anticipate preselected glucose levels and to warn of impending hypoglycaemia.

As far as the professional segment is concerned, it is worth pointing out that professional continuous glucose monitoring (pCGM) has became a commonly accepted term for the use of continuous glucose testing supervised by healthcare professionals. With the advent of continuous monitoring devices for home use such as the FreeStyle Navigator [40, 41], a distinction between the two types of monitoring is needed. More specifically, pCGM is a 3–5 day test done to evaluate glucose control retrospectively, with the glucose results being unknown by the patient until the results are downloaded after the testing period. pCGM, often in use in ambulatories, out-patient clinics, anti-diabetic centres and hospital metabolic units, enables medical doctors and patients to evaluate the effects of diet, physical activity, medication and life style events over the course of 24 h or even longer. Microdialysis-based systems fit very well with the requirement of the professional segment (i.e. GlucoDay) [27], although also some needle-type devices such as Medtronic's Guardian are a good match with HCP needs [29]. Finally, regarding the critical care segment, a critical CGMS is a system specifically conceived for ICUs, which require quick turnaround times. Because in critical care time matters, the only way to eliminate lag time is to measure glucose directly in the blood stream. As such, these systems are equipped with central or peripheral catheters and employ as a measuring principle that of either microdialysis- or fluorescence-based glucose sensors or a similar principle known as a fluorescence resonance energy transfer (FRET) system. The latter technique has been implemented to limit the deterioration of commonly employed sensors, provided that a sensor inserted in the body of a critically ill patient would be replaced after 3 days.

From a clinical perspective, despite efforts to develop intravenous critical CGMSs for tight glycaemic control (TGC), this procedure in critically ill patients remains a highly controversial issue. The strict euglycaemic range of 80–110 mg/dL as proposed by Leuven trials (Greet Van Den Berghe) was criticised by more recent studies and particularly by the NICE-SUGAR study [82], which demonstrated an increased mortality in the intensive glucose control group (81–108 mg/dL) compared with conventionally treated patients (<180 mg/dL). Despite the outcomes of these studies, it is worth pointing out that an accurate and precise assessment of glycaemic variability is important and can be performed only using CGM. Finally, intravenous CGMSs allow ICU staff to assess the effects of diverse intensive insulin therapy schemes on patient glucose levels in real time. As such, critical CGM permits the execution of TGC protocols without fear of undetected hypoglycaemic events (Fig. 2.39).

Clinical Indications and Target Population

Although CGM provides a complete picture of a patient's glucose levels throughout the day, clinical applications have not yet been well established. In general, these systems can be particularly useful in determining patterns of glycaemia over the course of 24 h and in detecting hypoglycaemia occurring at night and unawareness. In fact, its ability to improve metabolic control has been demonstrated only in

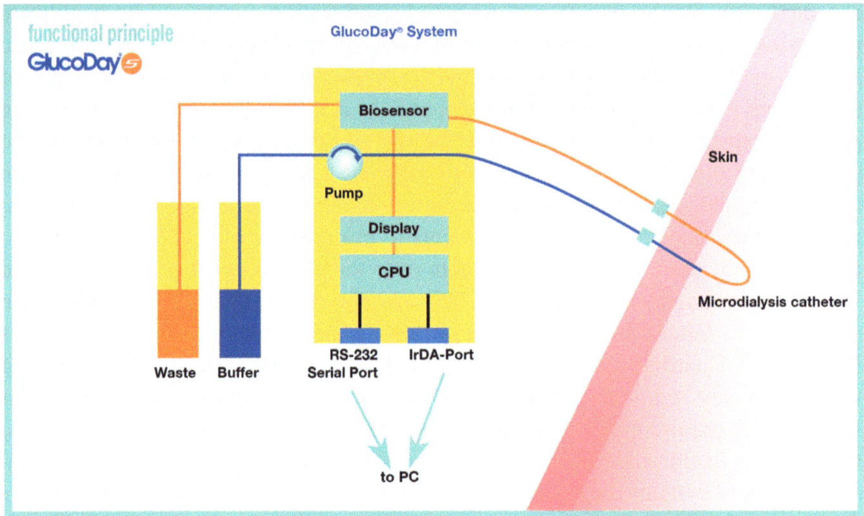

Fig. 2.39 Scheme of the glucoday functional principle

specific clinical scenarios. Nevertheless, although there are already several clinical indications for using CGM [30, 31, 39, 42, 46, 47], including:

1. Assessment of impact of insulin dosing and therapy adjustment to improve metabolic control;
2. Achievement of tighter glycaemic control without causing hypoglycaemia, especially in paediatric cases, gestational diabetes and critically ill patients treated in surgical and medical ICUs;
3. Diagnosis of hypoglycaemia unawareness and prevention of nocturnal hypoglycaemia.

As far as the target population is concerned, the desirable characteristics for using CGM are the same as those appropriate for insulin pump therapy. Individuals should possess mechanical dexterity, intelligence, reliability, knowledge of diabetes and commitment because they will be using sophisticated equipment. Moreover, patients need to understand the impact and duration of their insulin boluses in response to CGM data to avoid the risk of excess insulin dosage.

In conclusion, patients who might benefit from the use of CGM include the following:

1. Patients with brittle diabetes with poor metabolic control or high glucose variability,
2. Patients with a fear of hypoglycaemia,
3. Patients with gastroparesis,
4. Pregnant women,
5. Critically ill patients.

Practical Issues and Limitations of CGMS Use

There are still significant limitations to overcome for CGMSs to have a direct and dramatic impact on patient care. From an analytical perspective, for example, discrepancies between sensor signal and reference methods are not uncommon. This happens for two main reasons: the differences in glucose concentration between blood and ISF that can be compensated only by specifically conceived proprietary algorithms and the calibration procedure that must be conducted in vivo using as a reference method a traditional glucose meter that is intrinsically less accurate and precise than a lab reference method. Indeed, sensor calibration is a key issue in CGM. First of all, after application of a CGM device a first calibration can be performed only when the sensor signal is stable, and this can take between 2 and 10 h. Moreover, a CGMS needs to be recalibrated several times to achieve good accuracy because all sensors show a given amount of signal drift as a result of a reaction with a foreign body caused by the sensor or catheter. In this respect, several experts have demonstrated the advantage of the microdyalysis technique employed by the GlucoDay device (A.Menarini Diagnostics), which minimises foreign body reactions. Next, system accuracy depends on the technological and physiological lag time, which is device-specific and affected by (1) sampling frequency, (2) membrane pore size, (3) probe size and, if the system is microdialysis-based, (4) dialysis perfusion rate. Finally, it is important to perform calibrations only when discrepancies between blood and ISF are very low, such as before meals.

Last but not least, the subcutaneous inflammatory reaction caused by an implanted sensor can produce the so-called biofouling effect, which consists of the formation of a fibrous wall that prevents the implanted device from interacting with the surrounding tissue (fibrosis encapsulation). From an economical perspective, despite different systems for continuous glucose monitoring (CGM) are available on the European market, there is no unlimited reimbursement for CGM use in any European country. In some countries, reimbursement exists for certain clinical indications but reimbursement situations across Europe differ significantly. From the scientific and clinical perspective a number of randomized controlled trials have demonstrated the efficacy of real-time CGM versus self-monitoring of blood glucose, at least for hemoglobin A1c reduction. Nevertheless, according to many health care professionals and potential CGM users, national health services and health insurance organizations are still reluctant to reimburse CGM [83].

Continuous Glucose Monitoring Systems for Intensive Care Unit Patients

Medical and surgical patients managed in the intensive care units (ICU) of the hospital experience a high incidence of hyperglycaemia, hypoglycaemia and glycaemic variability despite significant hospital resources allocated to glucose control [60].

Table 2.11 Physico-chemical characteristics of a normal arterial blood sample

	Abbott Freestyle Navigator	DexCom SEVEN PLUS	Medtronic MiniMed Guardian REAL-Time	A. Menarini Diagnostics GlucoDay S	A. Menarini Diagnostics GMD
Detection	Amperometric (3-electrode system)	Amperometric (2-electrode system)	Amperometric (3-electrode system)	Amperometric (2-electrode system)	Amperometric (2-electrode system)
Working electrode	Carbon	Pt wire	Pt (plated on plastic)	Pt wire	Carbon (printed)
Reference electrode	Ag/AgCl	Ag/AgCl	Ag/AgCl (printed)	Ag/AgCl	Ag/AgCl (printed)
Counter electrode	Carbon	–	Pt (plated on plastic)	–	–
Mediator	OS-redox hydrogel	–	–	–	Prussian blue
System generation	Second (redox mediated)	First (H_2O_2 oxidation)	First (H_2O_2 oxidation)	First (H_2O_2 oxidation)	First (H_2O_2 reduction)
Operating potential versus Ag/AgCl	40 mV	500–700 mV	700 mV	620 mV	–20 mV
Enzyme	GOx (cross-linked Wired Enzyme™)	GOx (cross linked)	GOx	GOx (cross linked)	GOx (cross linked)
Flux modulating membrane	Cationic (vinyl pyridine-styrene copolymer)	Neutral (polyurethane/ polyethylene glycol copolymer)[a]	Neutral (polyurethane/ polyurea/polyethylene glycol/polysiloxane copolymer)[a]	Anionic (cellulose acetate/ polycarbonate)	Anionic (NAFION)

Oxygen dependence	Negligible	Moderate++	Moderate++	Moderate+	Moderate+
Microdialysis probe material	–	–	–	Regenerated cellulose	Polyethersulfone/polyvinyl pyrrolidone (subcutaneous probe); polyamide (intravascular probe)
Range of linear response	20–500 mg/dl	40–400 mg/dl	40–400 mg/dl	20–600 mg/dl	5–400 mg/dl
Insertion depth and angle	5 mm, 90°	12 mm, 45°	12 mm, 45°	~3–5 mm, ~0°	~3–5 mm, ~20°
Run-in time	10 h	2 h	2 h	2 h	2 h
Sensor lifetime	5 days (120 h)	7 days (166 h)	3 days (72 h)	2 days (48 h)	>4 days (100 h)
Data update frequency	1/min	1/5 min	1/5 min	1/3 min	1/min
Calibration frequency	After 10, 12, 24, 72 h	After 2 h; every 12 h thereafter	After 2, 6, 12 h; every 12 h thereafter	After 2 h; every 12 h thereafter	After 2 and 10 h; every 24 h thereafter

[a] Information obtained from patent literature; it may be inaccurate.

An increasing number of studies are confirming that high glycaemic variability represents an important outcome predictor in critically ill patients who develop stress-induced hyperglycaemia associated with several adverse outcomes that can increase mortality, morbidity and in-hospital stay [32, 33, 55]. As a matter of fact, clinicians are challenged to dose insulin at the optimal time according to changes in nutrient intakes, insulin sensitivity, hydration status and organ function (renal, hepatic, gastrointestinal and cardiovascular) [60]. Moreover, tight glycaemic control (TGC) is today performed in several ICUs and High Dependent Units (HDU) by taking and analysing blood sample every 30–60 min in order to maintain normoglycamia and avoid complications such as severe infections and multiple organ failures. However, TGC programs increase the nursing workload and its implementation may result in a challenge as it requires a change in the established practice as well as an adequate training of the nursing staff. The application of CGMs in ICUs is a promising tool for reducing medical staff efforts while providing real-time information on both the absolute value and the trend of blood glucose concentration levels. Even though a number of CGMSs are now available on the market, their use in ICU settings is still very limited due primarily to the fact that most CGMSs currently available operate in the ISF, whereas treatment protocols are essentially based on venous blood (VB) glucose values. Between the ISF and the VB glucose values a time lag exists that can change depending on a number of factors, including hypotension or therapeutic treatment, which can significantly reduce the correlation between these two components in the case of rapid glucose fluctuations. Moreover, after conditions of shock, oedema or anaerobic glucose utilisation, the correlation between the two components might significantly and unpredictably decrease. This would suggest that the development of a CGMS capable of operating directly in VB could overcome any remaining problems still limiting the application of CGMSs in ICUs. Although in the intensive care market dedicated CGMSs for critically ill patients are not yet commercially available, several devices have been proposed, developed and finally tested, as previously mentioned. Generally, they exploit an existing central or peripheral intravascular line for the insertion of a specific catheter for direct blood sampling, microdialysis or for the housing of the sensor itself (e.g. a miniaturised fibre-optic platform) [25–27]. Various technologies have been investigated for glucose detection: near-infrared spectroscopy, fluorescence, and enzyme-based biosensors. Three systems, OptiScanner (OptiScan Biomedical, Hayward, California, US), Eirus (Maquette, Rastatt, Germany) and GlucoClear (Dexcom/Edwards, Irvine, California, US) have been CE marked (Fig. 2.40). The former is a plasma-based bedside glucose monitoring system that draws small amounts (120 μL) of patient blood every 15 min, converts the blood into plasma and then transports the sample to be read by a near-infrared spectrometer [52]. Eirus is a system based on a specific microdialysis central venous catheter able to collect small metabolites like glucose and lactate, which are measured at regular intervals by an enzyme-based biosensor. As already discussed, Microdialysis is a technique where a cather with a semipermeable membrane is perfused with a dialysis fluid. When inserted in a vein, the dialysis fluid in the microdialysis catheter equilibrates with the small molecules in plasma to be measured. Measurements of these molecule in

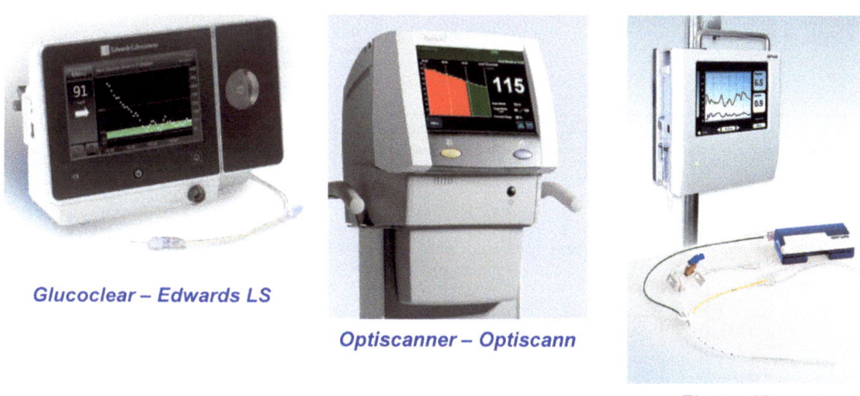

Fig. 2.40 Intravascular CGMs with CE mark

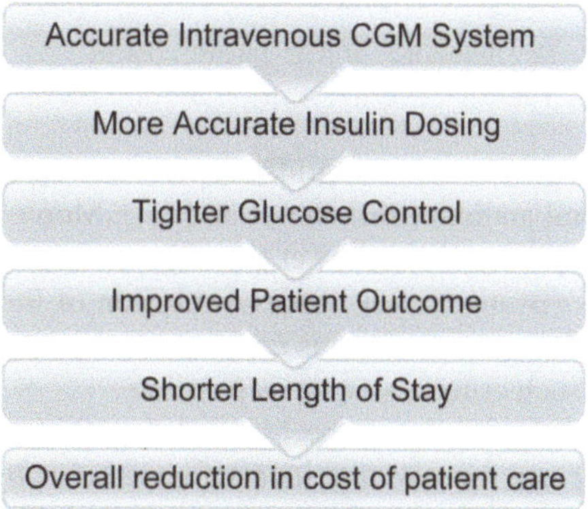

Fig. 2.41 The Cascade of benefits of accurate Glucose measurement in ICU

the dyalisate represent their concentration in plasma. Moreover, because no blood samples are needed, this technique can give continuous readings of plasma glucose values [53, 66]. GlucoClear is a bedside glucose monitoring system that draws small amounts of patient blood and then transports the sample to be read by an external GOx glucose biosensor [28]. Other systems (e.g. GlySure, Glumetrix) have been presented in various sector-specific assemblies, but their clinical validation is still in progress. Regarding the therapeutic impact of inaccuracies in the reading of blood glucose concentrations (see in Fig. 2.41 the cascade effects of measurement accuracy), error grids adaptable to the actual insulin algorithms that are used in ICUs are needed.

In fact, the current Clarke error grid was developed to assess the performance of intermittent glucose meters in diabetics, but it has not been adapted for use in

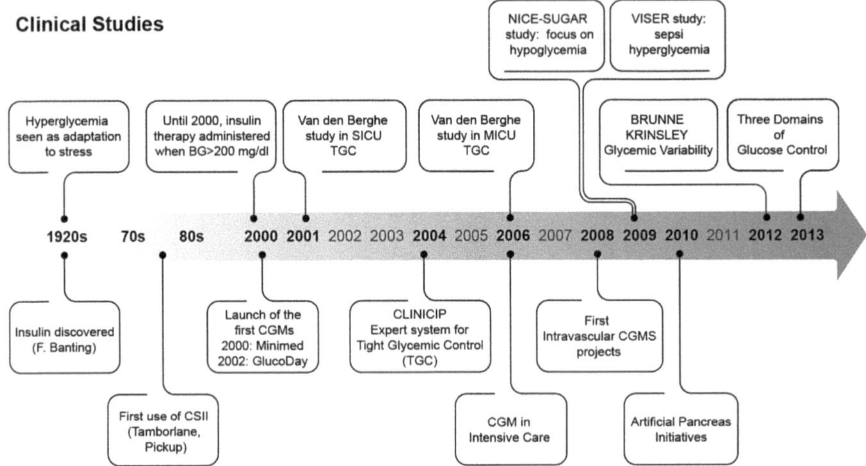

Fig. 2.42 Key milestones of ICU glucose control

ICUs. In particular, error grids adapted to an actual target range have been published by several authors (Ellmerer et al. [81]). Moreover, error grids for CGM have also been proposed (Kovatchev et al. [80]) and used to assess the impact of inaccuracies in ICUs (Brunner et al. [85]). A revision of the required criteria for clearance by the regulatory authorities is currently under way, and many experts are working to release such criteria as soon as possible.

To conclude, it may be asserted that CGMSs in ICUs are expected to be the next big step forward in critical care medicine by permitting the implementation of accurate and effective TGC procedures in the SICU and MICU settings. However, despite this promises, continuous glucose monitoring systems for ICU applications presently lack standardisation. Therefore, in 2012 a meeting of 16 experts plus invited observers from industry was organised to discuss and where possible reach consensus on the most appropriate methods to measure and monitor blood glucose in critically ill patients and on how glycaemic control should be assessed and reported. Recommendations covered many different areas (i.e. appropriate performance standards, sampling frequency, methods and technology, etc.) and are now available in a specific paper published in the journal "Critical Care" on 2013 [64]. Figure 2.42 reports a schematic representation of advances in clinical and technical progression that led to the present consensus on the need for ICU glucose control. As stated by Rice and Cursin (2012) "the question of whether outcome will be improved by maintaining BG within a narrow range can only be answered when rapid, accurate, interference free, inert and cost-effective CGM systems are validated for clinical use". In view of the present clinical and technological trends in critical care [50, 54, 58, 59], and despite the current uncertainties regarding the optimal blood glucose levels to be achieved in critically ill patients, there is no doubt that the combination of CGMSs and insulin algorithms represent promising tools that will enable clinicians to avoid the three domains of dysglycaemia associated with increased mortality and will lead the way towards a computer-assisted insulin delivery system, also known as an artificial pancreas [56, 57].

Fully Implantable Biosensors

An alternative approach to the traditional CGMS is the total implantation of a glucose-sensing device with subsequent non-invasive measurements from outside the body. The main advantage of such a solution would be the absence of transcutaneous material: with this approach, glucose measurements can be discrete or continuous, depending on the technology. It is still under debate whether the implantation site should be in a blood vessel, with the risk of blood clotting, or in a subcutaneous tissue. The subcutaneous tissue seems to be more appropriate because it is relatively surgically accessible; however, various authors have pointed out that both the life cycle and the reliability of a sensor implanted in such a site are very limited. One of the major obstacles to the implementation of a commercial fully implantable biosensor is that none of the prototypes tested so far were capable of monitoring glucose for more than few hours due to a sensible signal drift caused by the aggressive inner environment. Moreover, most such prototypes were able to work properly once removed from the body and used in vitro, demonstrating that the biological environment plays a crucial role in the difficulties faced by implantable biosensors. There are several effects caused by biocompatibility issues, the most important of which is the build-up of tissue around the sensor as a result of its implantation. This affects diffusion to and from the sensors and results in readings that do not accurately reflect current blood glucose levels. A very recent study reported that adding an interfacing angiogenesis membrane stimulated the growth of capillaries around the sensor and improved sensor longevity and the dynamic range and stability of calibration. Surprisingly, the study pointed out that using the aforementioned approach, it was possible to monitor glucose in subcutaneous tissue in a wide temporal window, namely for more than 100 days. Some researchers are instead working on intravascular fully implantable sensors, and clinical trials have been started with such sensors. One caveat for both types is that some glucose-sensing molecules are toxic, and it is unclear whether regulatory authorities will accept the insertion of such implants, even if only a very small number are inserted and well covered.

Minimally Invasive and Non-Invasive Sensors

The disadvantages of currently available CGMSs are the relatively short life of the sensors (up to 7 days), the pain associated with the insertion of needles into subcutaneous tissue, the risk of infection and subsequent inflammation due to breaking the skin barrier, the poor quality of the measurements and the fact that glucose changes are monitored in the ISF and not directly in the blood stream. In addition, current CGMSs require calibration against blood glucose values as often as twice a day. Furthermore, many individuals with diabetes have the perception that CGM devices interfere with daily activities. A glucose monitor that could be worn discretely and removed when desired without requiring the inconvenience and cost of sensor replacement and recalibration would likely change perceptions for the better. In attempting to overcome at least part of this risk, some companies are developing minimally invasive CGMSs with improved functions using nanotechnology approaches. A different but very interesting sampling device was developed by Kumetrix (Union City, CA) based on silicon microneedles similar in size to human hair. The aim was to develop a handheld battery-powered electronic monitor that would accept a cartridge loaded with disposable sampling devices. Each disposable consists of a microneedle and a receptacle into which the blood sample is drawn. To take a measurement, the patient loads the cartridge into the electronic monitor and simply presses the monitor against the skin. This action will cause the microneedle to penetrate the skin and draw a very small volume of blood ($<$ 100 nL) into the disposable element, where the blood glucose concentration would be measured.

As for non-invasive devices, ideally the objective is to have a CGMS like a wristwatch or a cuff around the arm or an ear clip that could be used to monitor changes in glycaemia non-invasively for prolonged periods of time without having to break the skin barrier. The measuring principles proposed so far are reported as follows:

1. Near-infrared spectrometry (NIR)
2. Mid-infrared spectrometry (Mid-IR)
3. Temperature-modulated localised reflectance
4. Polarimetric techniques
5. Ultrasound technology
6. Fluorescence techniques
7. Thermal spectroscopy
8. Impedance spectroscopy
9. Electromagnetic sensing and radio-frequency spectroscopy
10. Optical analysis through the eye (i.e. spectral analysis of the chemical components in the vitreous humour)
11. Iontophoresis

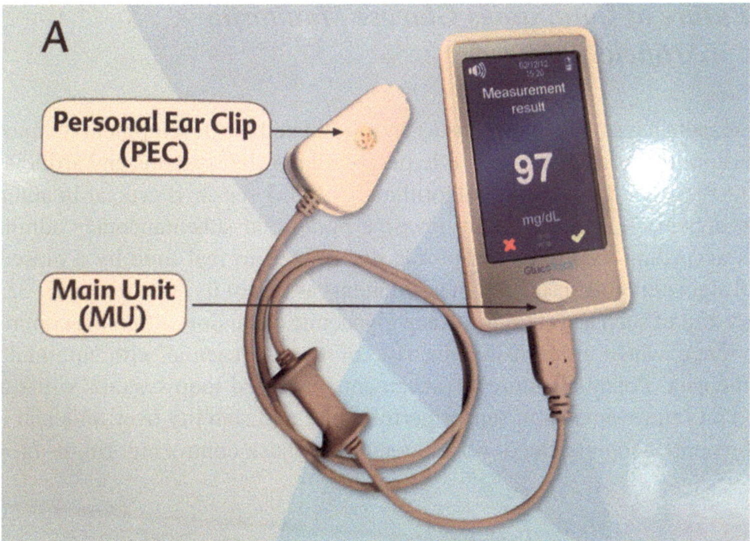

Fig. 2.43 Integrity's GlucoTrack

An interesting recently developed device is the Glucotrak (Fig. 2.43), which consists of an ear clip for glucose detection and a palm-sized unit for signal processing and data visualisation. Glucose is measured through multivariate regression analysis that converts ultrasonic, electromagnetic and thermal signals into a glucose concentration. The device is presented in the figure below.

Considerable progress has been made in the development of non-invasive glucose devices; however, at the time of writing, frequent testing using invasive blood glucose determination via finger-sticking provides the best information for diabetes disease management. Despite more or less regular announcements that a breakthrough has been achieved, despite more than 30 years of intensive work on non-invasive glucose sensors and the investment of at least US$1 or 2 billion, no system that allows non-invasive glucose monitoring in daily life with sufficient reliability is yet available. Most scientists are more sceptical than ever that it will be possible to monitor glucose non-invasively. Also, one of the most recent approaches, impedance spectrometry, developed by Carduff et al. in the Solianis Project, did not yield the expected results in terms of reliable monitoring of trends in glycaemia. Because a monitor that is accurate, continuous, non-invasive, non-intrusive, and possessing a sensor with a long life would undoubtedly increase the frequency of CGM use and empower individuals to assume more control over their diabetes, improving their health and quality of life, not surprisingly research continues in this area, and much effort is being devoted to developing such a monitor [61].

The Future of Continuous Glucose Monitoring and the Artificial Pancreas

CGM sensors have opened new vistas and stimulated the development of innovative on-line applications, such as hypo-/hyperglycaemia alert systems and artificial pancreas (AP) closed-loop control algorithms. A CGM sensor is crucial in automated insulin delivery, i.e. a minimally invasive pump that subcutaneously administers insulin according to a temporal profile determined in real time by a closed-loop control algorithm that has CGM measurements as one of its key inputs [33–38]. The primary aim of such a system is to keep glycaemic excursion within a recommended target range whilst minimising the risk of hypoglycaemia with minimal input from the user. Potential future advancements in closed-loop systems will strongly depend on improvements in sensor performance and stability over time and on the development of sophisticated, yet accurate and robust, control algorithms [43].

Conclusions

Biosensors are widely used in medicine to monitor or detect biological molecules for applications ranging from diabetes to cancer. Moreover the recent progresses in micro and nanoscale technologies will shortly permit to improve further their performances in terms of portability, cost-effectiveness, specificity, sensitivity, linear dynamic range and detection limits. At present, electrochemistry biosensors are one of the best options to provide low cost-technologies for measuring glucose, a substrate of paramount importance for the monitoring and treatment of diabetes mellitus. Therefore, the aim of this chapter was to provide an in-depth overview of the different sensing strategies to measure glucose, regardless if they were only proposed in literature or if they were afterword engineered and made commercially available by the industry. The principles and the detection mechanisms were explained and some commercial products were reported. Aside from intermittent glucose measurements, several paragraphs were dedicated to the CGM systems which are presently gaining spotlight within the medical community: in fact, the commercial glucose measurement market accounts for billions of dollars and CGM is rapidly tapping into this arena. CGM systems are increasingly used both in the management of individuals with type 1 diabetes, and for selected individuals with type 2 diabetes. These devices are now migrating to the perioperative environment and in the ICU settings: therefore anesthesiologists need to be familiar with them and know their limitations. Although CGMs (or the new generation of fully implantable sensors) may facilitate glucose control and insulin administration, the future lays in closed-loop systems consisting of computer-based algorithms guided by a CGM device in order to achieve the therapeutic goals. A successful system is likely to be nurse-centered, fully integrated into the routine workflow, transparent, equipped with feedback mechanisms, and based upon patient-specific information.

Closed-loop solutions, which might find a first widespread use in the controlled environment of the intensive care units and afterword spin-off to other areas, can give a key contribution in altering the current clinical practices, thus introducing a new concept, referred to as "High-Tech/High-Touch Medicine".

Acknowledgement The authors wish to thank Dr. Andrei Malic, European Director of Medical and Scientific Affairs, at Nova Biomedical Corporation (Waltham, MA, USA) for his constructive comments on the paragraph related to the hospital point of care systems and for his helpful scientific support to all the analytical and clinical studies on POCT devices carried-out together.

References

1. Wang J., 2008. Electrochemical glucose biosensors, Chem. Rev., 108, 814–825.
2. Reach. G.; Wilason G.S., 1992. Anal. Chem. 64, 381A.
3. P. D'Orazio, R.W. Burnett, N. Fogh-Andersen, E. Jacobs, K. Kuwa, W.R. Kulpmann, L. Larsson, A. Lewenstam, A.H.J. Maas, G. Mager, J.W. Naskalski, A.O. Okorodudu, 2005. Clin. Chem. 51, 1573–1576.
4. Frank M Brunkhorst and Hans G Wahl.Blood glucose measurements in the critically ill more than just a blood draw. Critical Care 2006, 10:178.
5. Kaplan L.A., Pesce A.J., Clinical Chemistry – Theory, analysis and correlation, 3rd Edition, 1996, Mosby-Year Book, Inc.
6. Price C. Point-of-care testing in diabetes mellitus. Clinic Chem Lab Med 41 1213–1219, 2003.
7. Tsuge, H., Natsuakai, O., and Ohashi, K. (1975). *J. Biochem.* **78**, 835–843.
8. J. Raba and H.A. Mottola, 1995. Glucose oxidase as an analytical reagent. *Critical Rev. Anal. Chem.*, 25, 1–42.
9. Swoboda, B. E. P. (1965) *Biochim. Biophys. Acta* **175**, 365–369.
10. Tsujimura S., Kojima S., Kano K., Ikeda T., Sato M., Sanada H., Omura H., 2006. Novel FAD-dependent glucose dehydrogenase for a dioxygen-insensitive glucose biosensor. *Biosci. Biotechnol. Biochem.* **70**, 654–659.
11. A. Heller and B. Feldman, 2008. Electrochemical Glucose Sensors and Their Applications in Diabetes Management. *Chem. Rev.* 108, 2482–2505.
12. Sode, K., Kojima, K., 1997. Improved substrate specificity and dynamic range for glucose measurement of *Escherichia coli* PQQ glucose dehydrogenase by site directed mutagenesis. Biotechnol. Lett. 19, 1073–1077.
13. J.G. Hauge, 1964. Glucose Dehydrogenase of Bacterium anitratum: an Enzyme with a Novel Prosthetic Group. J. Biol. Chem. 239, 3630–3639.
14. Karp G., Cell and Molecular Biology, 5th Ed., Wiley, 2008.
15. Loach P.A., 1976. In *Handbook of Biochemistry and Molecular Biology*, 3rd ed. (Fasman, G.D., ed.), *Physical and Chemical Data*, vol. 1, pp. 122–130, CRC Press, Boca Raton, FL.
16. Duine, J.A., Frank, J., van Zeeland, J.K., 1979. Glucose dehydrogenase from *Acinetobacter calcoaceticus*: a 'quinoprotein'. FEBS Lett. 108, 443–446.
17. Ling. Ye, Martin. Haemmerle, Arjen J. J. Olsthoorn, Wolfgang. Schuhmann, Hans Ludwig. Schmidt, Johannis A. Duine, Adam. Heller. High current density "wired" quinoprotein glucose dehydrogenase electrode. *Anal. Chem.*, **1993**, *65* (3), pp 238–241.
18. http://www.amano-enzyme.co.jp/pdf/wave_e/vol10/vol10e_p2.pdf
19. http://www.amano-enzyme.co.jp/pdf/wave_e/vol5/vol5_topic.pdf
20. Prof. L. Laffel, personal communication.
21. Nicolas Mano and Adam Heller. Detection of Glucose at 2 fM Concentration. *Anal. Chem.*, **2005**, *77*, 729–732.
22. Tang Z, Du X, Louie RF, Kost GJ : Effects of drugs on glucose measurements with handheld glucose metes and a portable glucose analyser. Am J Clin Pathol 113: 75–86, 2000.

23. NCCLS Guideline EP7-P, Interference Testing in Clinical Chemistry.
24. Witt et al., 2000. Biochem. J. 347, 553–559.
25. Tang Z, Du X, Louie RF, Kost GJ : Effects of pH on glucose measurement with handheld glucose meters and portable glucose analyser for point-of-care testing. Arch Pathol Lab Med 124:577–582, 2000.
26. B. Innocenti, F. Mastrantonio, "POCT and connectivity: towards the laboratory without boundaries". *Hospital Healthcare Europe*, 2005/20 06, L15-L17
27. Maran A., Crepaldi C., Tiengo A., Grassi G., Vitali E., Pagano G., Bistoni S. et al. Continuous subcutaneous glucose monitoring in diabetic patients: a multicenter analysis. *Diabetes Care* **25**: 347, 2002.
28. Wentholt I.M., Volle Bregt M.A., Hart A.A., Hoekstra J.B., DeVries J.H. Comparison of a needle-type and a microdialysis Continuous Glucose Monitoring in Type 1 Diabetic Patients. *Diabetes Care* **28**: 2871, 2005.
29. Kovatchev B., Anderson S., Heinemann L., Clarke W. Comparison of the Numerical and Clinical Accuracy of Four Continuous Glucose Monitors. *Diabetes Care* **31**: 1160, 2008.
30. Mello G., Parretti E., Tondi F., Bruno S., Iannuzzi L., DiCianni G., La polla A., Messeri D., Poscia A., Correlations between post-prandial glucose areas measured by continuous glucose monitoring (GlucoDay®) and fetal body composition in pregnant women with normal glucose tolerance. *Am. J. Obstet. Gynecol.* **193**: S90, 2005.
31. De Block C., Keenoy B.M., VanGaal L., Rogiers P., Intensive insulin therapy in the intensive care unit: assessment by continuous glucose monitoring. *Diabetes Care* **29**: 1750, 2006.
32. Van Den Berghe G., Wouters P., Weekers F., Verweast C. Intensive Insulin Therapy in Critically ill Patients. *N. Engl. J. Med.* **345**: 1359, 2001.
33. Van den Berghe G., Wilmer A., Hermans G., Meersseman W., Wouters P.J., Milants I., Van Wijngaerden E., Bobbaers H., Bouillon R. Intensive insulin therapy in the medical ICU. *N. Engl. J. Med.* **354**: 449, 2006.
34. Pfeiffer E.F., Thum C., Clemens A. The artificial beta cell. A continuous control of blood sugar by external regulation of insulin infusion. *Horm. Metabol. Res.* **6**: 339, 1974.
35. Fogt E.J., Dodd L.M., Jenning E.M., Clemens A.H. Development and evaluation of a glucose analyzer for a glucose-controlled insulin infusion system (Biostator®). *Clin. Chem.* **24**(8): 1366, 1978.
36. Keenan D.B., Cartaya R., Mastrototaro J.J. Accuracy of a New Real-Time Continuous Glucose Monitoring Algorithm. *J. Diabetes Sci. Technol.* **4**(1): 111, 2010.
37. Bode B., Gross K., Rikalo N., Schwartz S., Wahl T., Page C., Gross T., Mastrototaro J.J. Alarms based on real time sensor glucose values alert patients to hypo and hyper glycemia: the Guardian Continuous Monitoring System. *Diabetes Technol. Ther.* **6**: 105, 2004.
38. Mastrototaro J.J., Shin J., Marcus A., Sulur G. The Accuracy and Efficacy of Real-Time Continuous Glucose Monitoring Sensor in Patients with Type 1 Diabetes. *Diabetes Technol. Ther.* **10**(5): 385, 2008.
39. Blevins T.C. Professional Continuous Glucose Monitoring in Clinical Practice 2010. *J. Diabetes Sci. Technol.* **4**(2): 440, 2010.
40. Weinstein R.L., Bugler J.R., Schwartz S.L., Peyser T.A., Brazg R.L., McGarraugh G.V. Accuracy of the 5-Day FreeStyle Navigator Continuous Glucose Monitoring System. *Diabetes Care* **30** (5): 1125, 2007.
41. McGarraugh G., Bergenstal R. Detection of hypoglycemia with continuous interstitial and traditional blood glucose monitoring using the FreeStyle Navigator Continuous Glucose Monitoring System. *Diabetes Technol. Ther.* **11**(3): 145, 2009.
42. Garg S., Jovanovic L. Relationship of fasting and hourly blood glucose levels to HbA1c values: safety, accuracy, and improvements in glucose profiles obtained using a 7-day continuous glucose sensor. *Diabetes Care* **29**(12): 2644, 2006.
43. Kamath A., Mahalingham A., Brauker J. Analysis of time lags and other sources of error of the DexCom SEVEN continuous glucose monitor. *Diabetes Technol. Ther.* **11**(11): 689, 2009.
44. Poscia A., Mascini M., Moscone D., Luzzana M., Caramenti G., Cremonesi P., Valgimigli F., Bongiovanni C., Varalli M. A microdialysis technique for continuous subcutaneous glucose monitoring in diabetic patients (part 1). *Biosens. Bioelectron.* **18**: 891, 2003.

45. Varalli M., Marelli G., Maran A., Bistoni S., Luzzana M., Cremonesi P., Caramenti G., Valgimigli F., Poscia A. A microdialysis technique for continuous subcutaneous glucose monitoring in diabetic patients (part 2). *Biosens. Bioelectron* **18**: 899, 2003.
46. De Block C., Vertommen J., Manuel-y-Keenoy B., Van Gaal L. Minimally-invasive and non-invasive continuous glucose monitoring systems: indications, advantages, limitations and clinical aspects. *Curr. Diabetes Rev.* **4**(3): 159, 2008.
47. Hermanns N., Kulzer B., Gulde C., Eberle H., Pradler E., Patzelt-Bath A., Haak T. Short-term effects on patient satisfaction of continuous glucose monitoring with the GlucoDay with real-time and retrospective access to glucose values: a crossover study. *Diabetes Technol. Ther.* **11**(5): 275, 2009.
48. Anke Sieg, Richard H. Guy, M. Begoña Delgado-Charro: Non-invasive Glucose monitoring by reverse iontophoresis in vivo: Application of the internal standard concept. *Clin. Chem.* **50**(8): 1383, 2004.
49. Wentholt I.M.E., Hoekstra J.B.L., Zwart A., DeVries J.H. Pendra goes Dutch: lessons for the CE mark in Europe. *Diabetologia* **48**: 1055, 2005.
50. Valgimigli F., Lucarelli F., Scuffi C., Morandi S., Sposato I. Evaluating the clinical accuracy of GlucoMen®Day: a novel microdialysis-based continuous glucose monitor. *J. Diabetes Sci. Technol.* **4** (5): 1182, 2010.
51. Peyser T., Zisser H., Khan U., Jovanovic L., Bevier W., Romey M., Suri J., Strasma P., Tiaden S. Gamsey S., Use of a novel fluorenscent glucose sensor in volunteer subjects with Type 1 Diabetes Mellitus *J. Diabetes Sci. Technol.* 5(3): 687, 2011.
52. Jax T., Heise T., Nosek L., Gable J., Lim G., Calentine C. Automated Near-Continuous Glucose Monitoring Measured in Plasma Using Mid-Infrared Spectroscopy *J. Diabetes Sci. Technol.* **5**(2): 345, 2011.
53. Möller F., Liska J., Eidhagen F., Franco-Cereceda A. Intravascular Microdialysis as a Method for Measuring Glucose and Lactate during and after Cardiac Surgery *J. Diabetes Sci. Technol.* **5**(5): 1099, 2011.
54. Lucarelli F., Ricci F., Caprio F., Valgimigli F., Scuffi C., Moscone D., Palleschi G. GlucoMen Day continuous glucose monitoring system: a screening for enzymatic and electrochemical interferents *J. Diabetes Sci. Technol.* **6**(5): 1172, 2012.
55. The Effect of Intensive Treatment of Diabetes on the Development and Progression of Long-Term Complications in Insulin-Dependent Diabetes Mellitus, The Diabetes Control and Complications Trial (DCCT) Research Group, *N Engl J Med* 1993; 329
56. Sparacino G., Zanon M., Facchinetti A., Zecchin C., Maran A. Cobelli C. Italian Contributions to the Development of Continuous Glucose Monitoring Sensors for Diabetes Management *Sensors* **2012**, *12*, 13753–13780
57. M.J. Rice, D.B. Coursin Continuous Measurement of Glucose - Facts and Challenges., *Anesthesiology* 116 (1), 199, 2012
58. J.-C. Preiser, The Future of Glucose Control in the ICU. *ICU Management*, 13 (1), 24. 2013
59. J.S. Krinsley et al., Diabetic status and the relation of the three domains of glycemic control to mortality in critically ill patients: an international multicenter cohort study. *Crit. Care* 17, R37, 2013.
60. Jeffrey I Joseph, D.O. Analysis: New Point-of-Care Blood Glucose Monitoring System for the Hospital Demonstrates Satisfactory Analytical Accuracy Using Blood from Critically Ill Patients—An Important Step toward Improved Blood Glucose Control in the Hospital Journal of Diabetes Science and Technology Volume 7, Issue 5, September 2013
61. J. Newman A, Turner Home blood glucose biosensors: a commercial perspective Biosensors & Bioelectronics (20) 2005 2435–2453
62. N.S. Oliver et al. Glucose sensors: a review of current and emerging technology Diabetic Medicine 2009 26, 197–210
63. D. Zahn et al. Novel device for quick measurement of glucose in POCT areas without pre-analytical steps based on multi-way glucose biosensor, Eng. Life Sci. 2009, 9 n. 5, 398–403
64. Simon Finfer, Jan Wernerman, Jean-Charles Preiser, Tony Cass, Thomas Desaive, Roman Hovorka, Jeffrey I Joseph, Mikhail Kosiborod, James Krinsley MD, Iain Mackenzie, Dieter Mesotten, Marcus Schulz, Mitchell G. Scott, Robert Slingerland, Greet Van den Berghe, Tom

Van Herpe, Consensus Recommendations on "Measurement of Blood Glucose and Reporting Glycemic Control in Critically Ill Adults" Critical Care 2013, 17: 229

65. Kaczmarek E, Guerra E, Mosca A, Mastrantonio F, Lucarelli F, Valgimigli F, Ceriotti F, "Comparative assessment of the performances of the StatStrip point-of-care testing device for the measurements of ketone bodies.", Biochimica Clinica, 2013, vol. 37, SS S683.
66. Rooyackers O., Blixt P, Wernerman J, "Continuos glucose monitoring by intravenous microdyalysis: influence of membrane length and dialysis flow-rate", Acta Anesthesiol.Scand., 2012
67. Tang Z, Louie R, Payes M, Chang K, Kost G: Oxygen effects on glucose measurements with a reference analyzer and three handheld meters. Diabetes Technol Ther 2000, 2:349–362
68. Tang Z, Du X, Louie R, Kost G: Effects of pH on glucose measurements with handheld glucose meters and a portable glucose analyzer for point-of-care testing. Arch Pathol Lab Med 2000, 124:577–582
69. Chance J, Li D, Jones K, Dyer K, Nichols J: Technical evaluation of five glucose meters with data management capabilities. Am J Clin Path 1999, 111:547–556
70. Louie R, Tang Z, Sutton D, Lee J, Kost G: Point-of-care glucose testing. Arch Pathol Lab Med 2000, 124:257–266
71. Tang Z, Lee J, Louie R, Kost G: Effects of different haematocrit levels on glucose measurements with handheld meters for point-of-care testing. Arch Pathol Lab Med 2000, 124:1135–1140
72. Boyd JC, Bruns DE. Quality specifications for glucose meters: assessment by simulation modeling of errors in insulin dose. Clin Chem 47: 209–14 (2001)
73. Mann E, Salinas J, Pidcoke H et al Error rates resulting from Anemia can be corrected in multiple commonly used point of care glucometers J Trauma 2008 64:15 – 21.
74. Krinsley J, Grover A. Severe hypoglycaemia in critically ill patients: risk factors and outcomes. Crit Care Med 2007; 35: 2262–2267
75. C.L.S.I., Point of care blood glucose testing in acute and chronic care facilities; approved guideline - Third edition. POCT12-A3. 2013. 33(2)
76. Karon B Griemann L Scott R et al Evaluation of the Impact of Haematocrit and Other Interference on the Accuracy of Hospital-Based Glucose Meters. Diabetes Technology & Therapeutics 2008 10, Number 2, 111–120
77. Holtzinger C Szelag, E. DuBois, et al. Evaluation of a New POCT Bedside Glucose Meter and Strip With Haematocrit and Interference Corrections Point of Care 2008 7, Number 1 1–6.
78. Hopf S, Graf, B., and Gruber, M Comparison of Point-of-Care Testing Glucose Results from Intensive Care Patients Measured with Network-Ready Devices, Diabetes Technology & TherapeuticsVolume 13, Number 10, 2011
79. International Organization for Standardization (ISO). In vitro diagnostic test systems. Requirements for blood-glucose monitoring systems for self-testing in managing diabetes mellitus. International Standard ISO 15197:2013
80. Kovatchev et al. Evaluating the accuracy of continuous glucose-monitoring sensors: continuous glucose–error grid analysis illustrated by TheraSense Freestyle Navigator data. Diabetes Care. 2004;27:1922–1928
81. Ellmerer et al. Clinical evaluation of alternative-site glucose measurements in patients after major cardiac surgery. Diabetes Care. 2006;29(6):1275–1281.
82. The NICE-SUGAR Study Investigators. Intensive versus Conventional Glucose Control in Critically Ill Patients. N Engl J Med 2009; 360:1283–1297
83. L. Heinemann et al. Reimbursement for Continuous Glucose Monitoring: A European View Journal of Diabetes Science and Technology Volume 6, Issue 6, November 2012
84. Mastrantonio F., Valgimigli F., Grassi L., Cappa P., De Micheli G., Carrara S., "Comparative Performance of Different Nanostructured Electrochemical Sensors on Insulin Detection" BioNanoSci., 2013 3:285–288
85. Brunner R, Kitzberger R, Miehsler W, Herkner H, Madl C, Holzinger U., Accuracy and reliability of a subcutaneous continuous glucose-monitoring system in critically ill patients. Crit Care Med. 2011; 16:659–664

Chapter 3
Wireless System with Multianalyte Implantable Biotransducer

Christian Kotanen and Anthony Guiseppi-Elie

Introduction

Modern potentiostat technology is facilitating novel research in the field of biosensors [1–6], and translational research is dependent upon making efficient potentiostat systems for implantable biosensor devices [6–10]. The potentiostat continues to be a viable frontend instrument for biosensor technology because it allows several electrochemical modes of biotransducer interrogation. Among these are amperometry (constant voltage), voltammetry (a swept voltage), and coulometry (charge integration). For implantable amperometric biosensor systems to fulfill their desired functionality in the most efficient way possible, developers must devote special consideration to size (footprint), power management, telemetry capabilities, and signal processing. An implantable potentiostat may be discrete

C. Kotanen
Center for Bioelectronics, Biosensors and Biochips (C3B), Clemson University Advanced Materials Center, 100 Technology Drive, Anderson, SC 29625, USA
e-mail: ckotane@clemson.edu

Department of Bioengineering, Clemson University, Clemson, SC 29634, USA

A. Guiseppi-Elie (✉)
Center for Bioelectronics, Biosensors and Biochips (C3B), Clemson University Advanced Materials Center, 100 Technology Drive, Anderson, SC 29625, USA

Department of Bioengineering, Clemson University, Clemson, SC 29634, USA

Department of Chemical and Biomolecular Engineering, Clemson University, Clemson, SC 29634, USA

Department of Electrical and Computer Engineering, Clemson University, Clemson, SC 29634, USA

ABTECH Scientific, Inc., Biotechnology Research Park, 800 East Leigh Street, Richmond, VA 23219, USA
e-mail: guiseppi@clemson.edu

W. Burleson and S. Carrara (eds.), *Security and Privacy for Implantable Medical Devices*, DOI 10.1007/978-1-4614-1674-6_3,

or an application-specific integrated circuit and may be fully implanted or of the type where the biotransducer is implanted and the instrumentation is affixed externally to the subject/patient. Fully implantable systems are strongly favored over transcutaneous devices because they avoid the plurality of problems associated with serious infections [11]. The biofilm of infectious colonies, usually composed of biopolymers such as polysaccharides, proteins, and lipids, provides protection against immune cells and the penetration of antimicrobial agents [12]. Biofilms, once formed, display a complex arrangement of various extracellular components and secondary structures that confer resistance against conventional antibiotic therapies [13]. Multi-antibiotic resistance among bacteria that infect transcutaneous devices is a source of burden on patients and the healthcare system [14–17]. The US Centers for Disease Control and Prevention (CDC) estimates that approximately 500,000 surgical site infections occur annually in the United States [17–20]. Implantable systems minimize the potential for infections and enable observation of biological phenomena in a more natural, physiologically relevant state wherein subjects are able to move about freely while being monitored. A two-channel, two-terminal wireless potentiostat system, the Pinnacle Technology 8151 potentiostat, was previously considered for use in a minimally invasive biosensor system for the management of hemorrhage-associated trauma [9, 21]. In this work, we utilize model electrochemical cells to consider the merits and drawbacks of the 8151 potentiostat for use with a novel implantable biotransducer, the MDEA 5037 [22].

Methods

Components

The 8100-K1 fixed-frequency wireless dual potentiostat system was purchased from Pinnacle Technology (Lawrence, KS). The kit contained the Pinnacle 8151 wireless potentiostat, the programmer, and a receiver base station (Model 8106) with USB cables. Software for data acquisition was also included in the kit.

Accuracy Testing of Pinnacle 8151 Potentiostat System

The accuracy of the 8151 potentiostat was tested using discrete combinations of two model or "dummy" cells. These model cells served as a virtual device under test (VDUT) and were applied to the two available channels of the potentiostat. The model cells consisted of (i) a single resistor (R) of 10 MΩ as prescribed by the manufacturer and (ii) a parallel resistor-capacitor (RC) network of $R = 10$ MΩ and capacitor of 1 μF. The single-resistor VDUT models facile electrochemical reactions having large heterogeneous electron transfer rate constants. The complex RC cell models real electrochemical cells wherein the double layer capacitance sits in parallel with faradaic reactions [23]. Two identical resistor cells and two identical RC cells were acquired from Pinnacle Technology. Bias potentials of 0.5 V were applied to channels 1 and 2 during experimentation. Thirteen discrete configurations of R and RC were tested on the two channels of the 8151 potentiostat and the percentage error between the two channels was calculated for the response to model R or RC cells in the following manner:

$$\%Error = \frac{|I_{Ch1} - I_{Ch2}|}{I_{Ch2}} * 100$$

where I_{Ch1} and I_{Ch2} refer to the current response of channels 1 and 2, respectively. The telemetry distance of the 8151 potentiostat was determined in a laboratory setting. A resistor of 10 MΩ was connected to channel 1 of the potentiostat, and a bias potential of 0.5 V was applied. The potentiostat was moved away from the base station until a loss of signal was observed.

Results and Discussion

Footprint

The 8151 potentiostat can capture signals coming from biotransducers and wirelessly transmit two digitized signals on a 916 Hz band to a central base station that is interfaced to a computer via USB. Transmission may be maintained for up to 72 h straight using a 3 V lithium battery. The full system with battery weighs approximately 8.7 g with a footprint of approximately 8.2 mm^3. The device is sufficiently small to allow continuous measurement with an implanted biotransducer while maintaining a comfortable size and weight for small animals such as rats [24, 25] and fish [26, 27]. Having externalized electronics is the current modality for implantable biosensor systems using this potentiostat, much like other commercially available, subcutaneous glucose monitors [28].

Telemetric Performance

The 8151 and MDEA 5037 biosensor system, as seen in Fig. 3.1, was previously shown to have the capability to measure and record two analytes simultaneously at two applied potentials [21]. Preliminary studies on the performance of unmodified MDEA 5037 transducers were performed in solutions of 1:1 mixture of 1.0 mM ferrocyanide and 1.0 mM ferricyanide ($E^{\text{o}} = 0.76$ V versus Ag/AgCl). Current was observed as a function of concentration at room temperature (25°C). Electrochemical measurements were taken with both MDEA 5037 electrochemical cells simultaneously in a two-electrode configuration of an on-board working electrode

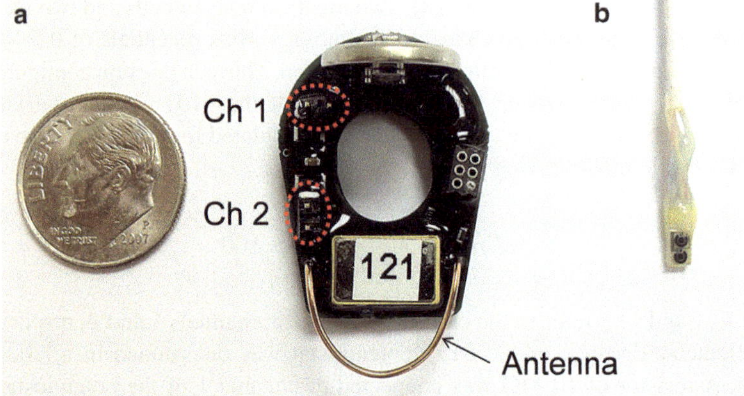

Fig. 3.1 Image of (**a**) the Pinnacle Technology 8151 wireless potentiostat showing the two channels with which it can interface with transducers such as (**b**) the MDEA 5037 implantable biochip with two independently addressable electrochemical cells, each having working, counter, and reference electrodes

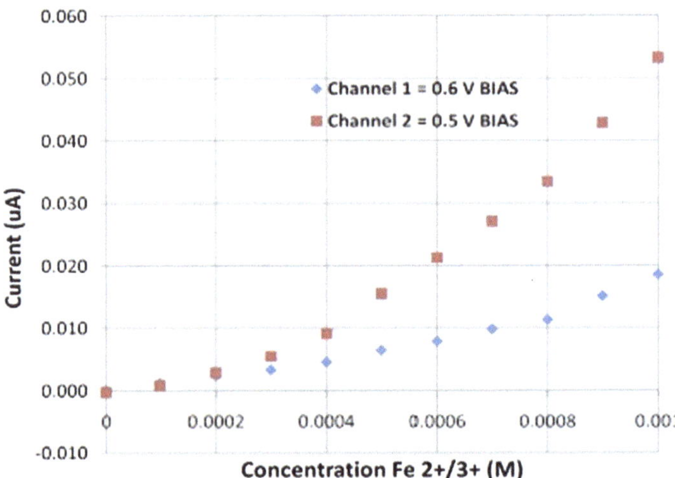

Fig. 3.2 An MDEA 5037 interfaced with the Pinnacle Technology 8151 potentiostat demonstrating the simultaneous measurement of Fe 2+/3+ at two different bias potentials applied to the two working electrodes of the MDEA 5037 [21]

array versus on-board counter electrode. Current was shown to monotonically increase as a function of ferri-/ferrocyanide at oxidative bias potentials of 0.5 (channel 1) and 0.6 V (channel 2) (Fig. 3.2). The equimolar, aqueous ferri-/ferrocyanide couple is an example of a facile electron transfer reaction with large heterogeneous rate constant at platinum. Calibration curves serve as sufficient evidence that current readings can be taken at different concentrations of solution and at different impressed potentials.

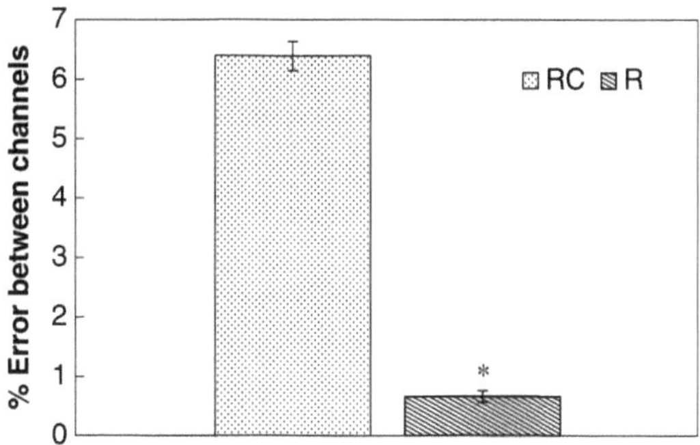

Fig. 3.3 The percentage error between channels of the Pinnacle Technology 8151 wireless potentiostat for complex (*RC*) and simple (*R*) circuits; 95% confidence intervals are shown (*denotes statistical significance from RC VDUTs with $p = 7 \times 10^{-8}$)

In a laboratory setting, the 8151 potentiostat maintained a steady and unbroken signal as far away as approximately 75 ft (23 m). If a line of sight to the base station was maintained, this distance could be increased to up to 100 ft (30 m) or more. The response time of the potentiostat was found to be between 2 and 8 s when performing amperometry. The overall performance makes this system advantageous for long-range monitoring of conscious animals in terms of footprint and telemetry performance. For future in vivo characterization, the biosensor system under development will have the biotransducer implanted in the trapezius muscle. Tunneling and exteriorization of lead wires will be necessary in order to interface with the potentiostat. Once the device is interfaced, interstitial glucose and lactate levels can be monitored remotely at an acquisition rate of 1 Hz.

Accuracy of Response of 8151 Potentiostat Channels

The current response of channels 1 and 2 to resistor (VDUT) cells averaged 49.9 (±0.1) nA and 49.6 (±0.0) nA ($n = 4$), respectively. The current response of channels 1 and 2 to the complex RC cell averaged 51.1 (±0.1) nA and 54.4 (±0.1) nA ($n = 6$), respectively. The percentage error between the two channels was determined to be 6.4 (±0.3) and 0.7 (±0.1) for RC and R model cells, respectively (Fig. 3.3). A two-tailed *t*-test indicated a significant difference in the mean percentage error when comparing the 8151 potentiostat response to R and RC circuits ($p \cong 10^{-8}$). These results indicate that the 8151 potentiostat system's two channels are within a reasonable 1% error for electrochemical redox reactions that are reversible and facile and can make reproducible results when using both channels simultaneously. A high level of reproducibility for this biosensor system has been observed during interrogation with ferrocene monocarboxylic acid (FcCOOH), a well-known redox mediator, which supports these findings [29].

For complex circuits using the resistor and capacitor in parallel, the 8151 system shows a large margin of error between the two channels. Ideally, the response from

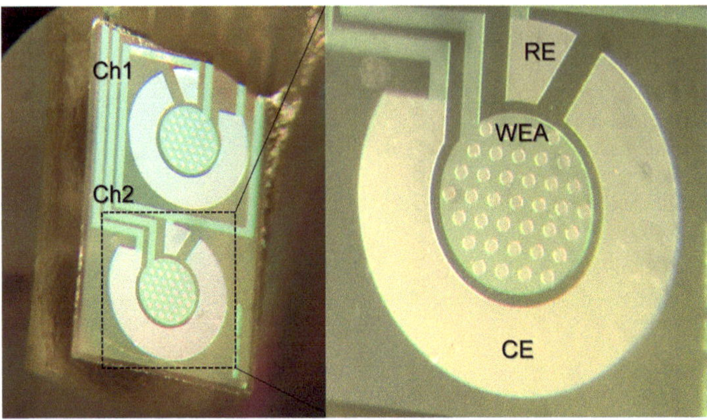

Fig. 3.4 Microscopic photograph of MDEA 5037 implantable transducer with two addressable cells that interface with the 8151 channels (channels 1 and 2); each cell has a working electrode array (*WEA*), counter electrode (*CE*), and reference electrode (*RE*)

both of the channels ought to be identical, much as was seen for the resistors tested. This difference in measurement will be problematic for complex electrochemical reactions such as during dual analyte sensing where both channels must be utilized simultaneously to monitor the analyte activity using two redox enzymes. We have established that the bias potentials applied by the 8151 to either of the two channels utilize a common reference, that is, the apparent four poles among the two channels are truly three poles. This means that during operation both of the independent counter/reference electrodes of each electrochemical cell share a single counter/reference electrode between the two independent working electrodes.

For clean MDEA 5037 transducers, having a common reference/counter electrode should not engender any significant changes to predicted chronoamperometric responses based on Cottrell's equation [30]. Current densities would be evenly distributed to both of the MDEA 5037 working electrodes during operation in simple electrochemical systems. For fully modified MDEA 5037 biotransducers with hydrogels, polypyrrole, and enzymes immobilized onto their microdisc array surfaces, current densities can be expected to be relatively uneven compared to the bare transducer. The design for the MDEA 5037 was with the intent to utilize each of its electrochemical cells (working, counter, and reference electrodes) independently (Fig. 3.4). An inability to do this will lead to unpredictable behavior between the two cells of the MDEA 5037. The full and independent characterization of all biotransducers fabricated will be necessary during future experimentation in vitro and in vivo when using the combined MDEA 5037 and the 8151 biosensor system. Unfortunately, additional biotransducer variability will now be introduced by the potentiostat system alone, which is less than ideal.

Wireless Security

The potentiostat wirelessly transmits packets of data to a base station using a radio frequency of 916 Hz. Wireless networks and technology have advanced around the world. The telemetry of patient information and data will advance along with diagnostic systems. For this reason it is important to protect data transmission in order to prevent the disclosure of confidential information. Wired Equivalent Privacy (WEP), Wi-Fi Protected Access (WPA), and 802.11i (WPA2) are among the common security mechanisms available. The general security mechanisms, however, will likely be insufficient for protecting confidential patient information. Some major weaknesses of WEP and WPA include their inability to prevent forgery of packets, allowing attackers to undetectably modify messages without knowing encryption keys, and allowing attackers to cause a denial-of-service attack if only some of layers of protection can be bypassed [31]. Security of WEP and WPA can be successfully breached within 10–20 min using a hacking utility such as Aircrack [31]. Security will be paramount for both military and civilian patient care.

Conclusions

The Pinnacle Technology 8151 wireless potentiostat was shown to have excellent response time and telemetric distance for small-animal testing. The potentiostat can communicate with a base station in a laboratory setting at a distance of up to 100 ft. The battery life is sufficient for continuous monitoring of up to 3 days, and the size/weight of the device makes it an excellent choice for biosensor animal models. The major drawback of the 8151 is its significant percentage of error between its two channels when measuring so-called real biosensors. A 6% error was observed between channels 1 and 2 for complex circuits. This inherent error could lead to inaccuracies during enzyme-based amperometric detection of analytes while using the two channels of the 8151 simultaneously. The MDEA 5037 transducer is a chip with two independently addressable electrochemical cells and could potentially be used with the 8151 potentiostat for performing dual analyte measurements. The two channels of the 8151 share a common reference/counter electrode and therefore require the independent working electrodes of the MDEA 5037 to utilize a common reference/counter electrode, contrary to its design. The 8151 dual potentiostat has excellent performance, aside from its lack of customizability. The design of the 8151 potentiostat would benefit greatly from options to allow the use of two independent reference/counter electrodes for the two channels of the potentiostat as well as sample and hold programming.

Acknowledgments This work was supported by the US Department of Defense (DoDPRMRP) Grant PR023081/DAMD17-03-1-0172, by the Consortium of the Clemson University Center for Bioelectronics, Biosensors and Biochips (C3B), and by ABTECH Scientific.

References

1. Beach, R.D., et al., *Towards a miniature implantable* in vivo *telemetry monitoring system dynamically configurable as a potentiostat or galvanostat for two- and three-electrode biosensors.* Instrumentation and Measurement, IEEE Transactions on, 2005. **54**(1): p. 61–72.
2. Yi-Fan, L., H. Chun-Yueh, and L. Bin-Da. *A Voltammetry Potentiostat Design for Large Dynamic Range Current Measurement.* in *Intelligent Computation and Bio-Medical Instrumentation (ICBMI), 2011 International Conference on.* 2011.
3. Frey, A., et al. *Digital potentiostat for electrochemical bio sensor chips.* in *ESSCIRC, 2010 Proceedings of the.* 2010.
4. Islam, A.B., et al. *A digitally controllable current readout circuit and modulator unit for remote monitoring and biotelemetry applications.* in *Electrical and Computer Engineering (ICECE), 2010 International Conference on.* 2010.
5. Chun-Yueh, H., et al. *A Portable Potentiostat with Molecularly Imprinted Polymeric Electrode for Dopamine Sensing.* in *Testing and Diagnosis, 2009. ICTD 2009. IEEE Circuits and Systems International Conference on.* 2009.
6. Razzaghpour, M., et al. *A highly-accurate low-power CMOS potentiostat for implantable biosensors.* in *Biomedical Circuits and Systems Conference (BioCAS), 2011 IEEE.* 2011.
7. Islam, A.B., et al. *A potentiostat circuit for multiple implantable electrochemical sensors.* in *Electrical and Computer Engineering (ICECE), 2010 International Conference on.* 2010.
8. Shuo, G., et al. *Wireless powered implantable bio-sensor tag system-on-chip for continuous glucose monitoring.* in *Biomedical Circuits and Systems Conference (BioCAS), 2011 IEEE.* 2011.
9. Guiseppi-Elie, A., *An implantable biochip to influence patient outcomes following trauma-induced hemorrhage.* Analytical and Bioanalytical Chemistry, 2011. **399**(1): p. 403–419.
10. Zhang, M., et al., *A low power sensor signal processing circuit for implantable biosensor applications.* Smart Materials & Structures, 2007. **16**(2): p. 525–530.
11. Donlan, R.M. and J.W. Costerton, *Biofilms: survival mechanisms of clinically relevant microorganisms.* Clin. Microbiol. Rev., 2002. **15**(2): p. 167–93.
12. Gotz, F., *Staphylococcus and biofilms.* Mol Microbiol, 2002. **43**(6): p. 1367–1378.
13. Gordon, R.J. and F.D. Lowy, *Pathogenesis of methicillin-resistant Staphylococcus aureus infection.* Clinical Infectious Diseases, 2008. **46**: p. S350-S359.
14. Fung, H.B., J.Y. Chang, and S. Kuczynski, *A practical guide to the treatment of complicated skin and soft tissue infections.* Drugs, 2003. **63**(14): p. 1459–80.
15. Horan, T.C., et al., *CDC definitions of nosocomial surgical site infections, 1992: a modification of CDC definitions of surgical wound infections.* Infect Control Hosp Epidemiol, 1992. **13**(10): p. 606–8.
16. Jawhara, S. and S. Mordon, In vivo *imaging of bioluminescent Escherichia coli in a cutaneous wound infection model for evaluation of an antibiotic therapy.* Antimicrobial agents and chemotherapy, 2004. **48**(9): p. 3436–41.
17. Kirkland, K.B., et al., *The impact of surgical-site infections in the 1990s: attributable mortality, excess length of hospitalization, and extra costs.* Infect Control Hosp Epidemiol, 1999. **20**(11): p. 725–30.
18. Bratzler, D.W. and P.M. Houck, *Antimicrobial prophylaxis for surgery: an advisory statement from the National Surgical Infection Prevention Project.* Clin Infect Dis, 2004. **38**(12): p. 1706–15.
19. Burke, J.P., *Infection control - a problem for patient safety.* N Engl J Med, 2003. **348**(7): p. 651–6.
20. Pharmacists, A.S.o.H.-S., *ASHP therapeutic guidelines on antimicrobial prophylaxis in surgery.* Am J Health-Syst Pharm., 1999. **56**: p. 1839–88.
21. Kotanen, C. and A. Guisepp-Elie, *Physiological Status monitoring for glucose and lactate during the onset of hemorrhagic shock.* American Society of Gravitational and Space Biology Bulletin, 2010. **23**(2): p. 55–63.

22. Rahman, A.R.A., G. Justin, and A. Guiseppi-Elie, *Towards an implantable biochip for glucose and lactate monitoring using microdisc electrode arrays (MDEAs).* Biomedical Microdevices, 2009. **11**(1): p. 75–85.
23. Franceschetti, D.R. and J.R. Macdonald, *Small-Signal A-C Response Theory for Electrochromic Thin Films.* Journal of The Electrochemical Society, 1982. **129**(8): p. 1754–1756.
24. Morita, H., et al., *Long-term hypergravity induces plastic alterations in vestibulo-cardiovascular reflex in conscious rats.* Neuroscience Letters, 2007. **412**(3): p. 201–205.
25. Wahono, N., et al., *Evaluation of permselective membranes for optimization of intracerebral amperometric glutamate biosensors.* Biosensors and Bioelectronics, 2012. **33**(1): p. 260–266.
26. Endo, H., et al., *Wireless enzyme sensor system for real-time monitoring of blood glucose levels in fish.* Biosensors and Bioelectronics, 2009. **24**(5): p. 1417–1423.
27. Endo, H., et al., *Wireless monitoring of blood glucose levels in flatfish with a needle biosensor.* Fisheries Science, 2010. **76**(4): p. 687–694.
28. Clarke, W.L., et al., *Closed-loop artificial pancreas using subcutaneous glucose sensing and insulin delivery and a model predictive control algorithm: the Virginia experience.* Journal of diabetes science and technology, 2009. **3**(5): p. 1031–8.
29. Kotanen, C. and A. Guiseppi-Elie, *Bioactive Electroconductive Hydrogels Yield Novel Biotransducers for Glucose.* Macromolecular Symposia, 2012.
30. Bard, A.J. and L.R. Faulkner, *Electrochemical Methods: Fundamentals and Applications.* Second Edition ed2001, New York: John Wiley & Sons.
31. Kumkar, V., et al., *Vulnerabilities of Wireless Security protocols (WEP and WPA2).* International Journal of Advanced Research in Computer Engineering & Technology (IJARCET), 2012. **1**(2): p. 34–38.

Chapter 4
New Concepts in Human Telemetry

Sandro Carrara

Personalized Therapy

Modern medicine is now facing a new challenge: personalizing the cures supplied to patients. This challenge relates to the main problem encountered in the past of low cure efficacy when providing pharmacological therapy to patients [1]. As schematically shown in Fig. 4.1, when a group of patients that have exactly the same disease is treated with exactly the same pharmacological compound (or a set of compounds), the result is usually four different types of patient responses: the best subgroup benefits from the cure with no toxic reaction; the second group benefits from the therapy but also experiences toxic reactions; the third subgroup experiences neither benefits nor toxic reactions; the fourth subgroup receives no benefit but, what is more, experiences severe toxic reactions.

This explains the extremely low success rates obtained in several therapies currently used against some of the most widespread diseases [1]. For example, only 25% of patients treated with highly aggressive drugs commonly used in chemotherapy get cancer recovered from the treatment, as shown in Table 4.1. On the other hand, cancer patients treated with anticancer compounds typically experience very clear toxic effects in areas of the body other than the location of the cancer. In this respect, the 25% rate of efficacy of cancer chemotherapy is surprisingly low. Society usually places its trust in pharmacological therapies based on overly simplified cases. For example, in the case of the flu (influenza), the illness is usually eliminated in all patients by simply using common antibacterial compounds. However, those compounds are not effective at all against virus attacks. In this case, the drugs simply minimize the side effects of bacterial infections that take place due to the weakness of the patient's immune system, which is fighting

S. Carrara (✉)
Schools of Engineering and Computer and Communication Science, École polytechnique fédérale de Lausanne, Lausanne, Switzerland
e-mail: Sandro.carrara@epfl.ch

W. Burleson and S. Carrara (eds.), *Security and Privacy for Implantable Medical Devices*,
DOI 10.1007/978-1-4614-1674-6_4, © Springer Science+Business Media New York 2014

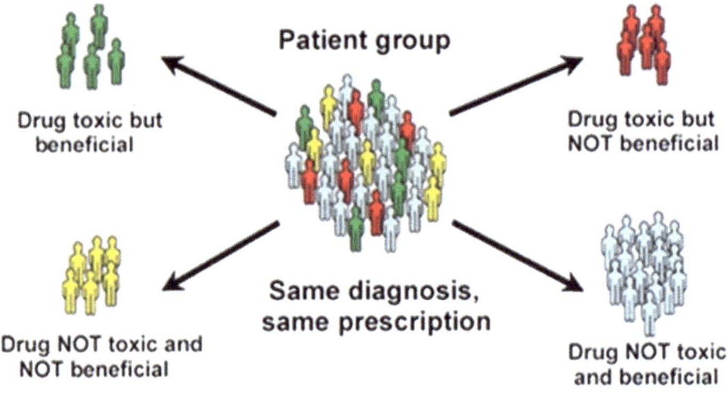

Fig. 4.1 Typical outputs from a group of patients treated with the same pharmacological therapy

Table 4.1 Rates of efficacy of standard pharmacological therapies

Therapeutic area	Rate of efficacy with standard drug treatment
Cancer (all types)	25%
Alzheimer's disease	30%
Incontinence	40%
Hepatitis C	47%
Osteoporosis	48%
Rheumatoid arthritis	50%
Migraine (prophylaxis)	50%
Migraine (acute)	52%
Diabetes	57%
Asthma	60%
Cardiac arrhythmias	60%
Schizophrenia	60%
Depression	62%

For depression, the data apply specifically to the drug class known as selective serotonin reuptake inhibitors.

Source: Brian B. Spear, Margo Heath-Chiozzi, and Jeffrey Huff, "Clinical Application of Pharmacogenetics," *Trends in Molecular Medicine* (May 2001).

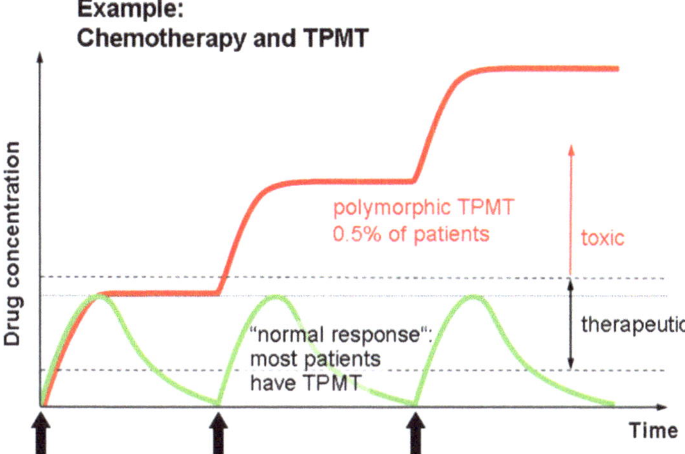

Fig. 4.2 Examples of dose trends in the case of patients with deleted (*red*) or not deleted (*green*) key metabolism enzymes

the viruses causing the flu. In contrast, a common situation in drug therapy is more like that of anticancer treatments, as summarized in Table 4.1.

Table 4.1 demonstrates that even very well-known and characterized diseases are not very treatable with pharmacological remedies. That is the case, for example, with diabetes. After several decades of medical research, the efficacy of drug compounds in the treatment of diabetes is no higher than 57%.

The reason for this low rate of efficacy in so many cases lies in the concept of biodiversity. Every patient is different with respect to all others, and thus it is tough to find a compound that shows 100% efficacy in all patients. To better understand the situation, consider the diversity among patients belonging to the same group. If we have a population of German patients and we must treat them all using the same drug compound, we need to consider that 7% of that population has deleted the genes of two key enzymes of human metabolism: the cytochromes P450 2D6 and 2C19 [2]. These proteins play a key role in metabolizing injected drug compounds and, in the case of gene deletion, the patient,s organism is no longer able to properly treat and expel the therapeutic molecule. For this reason, these patients show toxic concentrations in their blood after a few successive injections of the drug, as depicted in Fig. 4.2.

The market has already tried once to solve this problem by providing a chip based on microarray technology and capable of clustering patients into four main groups: ultrafast metabolizers, fast metabolizers, slow metabolizers, and ultraslow metabolizers [3]. However, the chip, produced by Roche, has not been very successful in the marketplace. The reason lies not in the chip, which is state of the art with respect to microarray technology, but in the nature of genetics. Patients differ not only at the level of gene expression but also at the level of gene regulation, epigenetics, and daily variations in their metabolism as well. Thus, oncologists have turned out to be not so interested in screening patients to cluster them by genetic predisposition. Oncologists are not interested in that because it does not prevent them from obtaining completely different, and in some cases adverse, outcomes from the same therapy on the same patient group.

One of the most recent and advanced approaches to addressing this problem is to attempt a full personalization of therapy on each individual patient [4]. The main idea here is to directly treat patients by monitoring their own personal parameters, both in terms of biomarkers related to the disease and in terms of the effective amount of supplied pharmacological compounds in the blood. That is, if a patient is given a drug compound in order to treat a disease that is marked by a specific molecule usually monitored in the blood, the idea might be to supply the right drug to the patient and then monitor the patient's blood with respect to the amount of the drug circulating as well as the amount of the disease marker. In practice, this is exactly what is usually done, typically three times per day, by patients suffering from diabetes mellitus type I. These patients have a pancreas that is no longer able to properly manage sugar levels in the blood (so-called glycemia/glycaemia) and therefore they require frequent insulin injections. Before deciding how much insulin to inject, these patients take a measure of their blood glucose values and then inject, with a syringe, the right amount of insulin required by that level of sugar. This is known as a control-feedback loop based on a measure of the disease marker and a corresponding injection of the proper amount of the required therapeutic compound. This control-feedback loop may be generalized to personalize the treatment for many well-known diseases requiring drug therapies. Moreover, a frequent (or continuous) monitoring of the drug amount in a patient's blood will help to avoid (or minimize) the risk of side effects due to toxic doses.

The Need to Monitor Several Metabolites

Implantable biosensors have attracted increased interest over the last 20 years. Since the appearance of the first publications [5] till the most recent devices in the market [6], tremendous efforts have been devoted to designing, fabricating, testing, and commercializing implantable biosensors. Several kinds of sensors have been fabricated to obtain implantable medical devices (IMDs). For example, pressure [7] and temperature [8] sensors and devices for glucose [6] and lactate [9] monitoring have appeared in the literature.

Over the last 20 years, implantable pumps have increasingly gained interest as well [10]. The literature contains reviews of both insulin pumps for diabetic patients [11] and devices for drug infusions for continuous release of chemotherapy compounds [12]. In more recent years, the concepts of implantable pumps and sensors have been combined to obtain implantable closed-loop systems for both glucose sensing and insulin delivery [13]. This idea can be generalized and extended to obtain artificial organs by monitoring human metabolism and providing artificial physiological regulation in an automatic manner. In fact, human metabolism

Table 4.2 Correlation between probe enzymes and commonly considered disease biomarkers (endogenous metabolites) and drugs (exogenous metabolites)

Probe enzyme	Endogenous metabolite	Exogenous metabolite
Glucose oxidase	Glucose	
Lactate oxidase	Lactate	
Glucose oxidase/hexokinase	ATP	
Cholesterol oxidase	Cholesterol	
P450 2B4		Benzphetamine
P450 3A4		Dextromethorphan
P450 3A4		Cyclophosphamide
P450 2C9		Flurbiprofen
P450 2C9		Naproxen

involves much more than simply monitoring glycemia and supplying the right amount of insulin. Even though a device for glucose monitoring/insulin release was the first closed-loop device proposed mainly for the diabetes market, an artificial pancreas would have to measure several other molecules besides glucose and provide several other molecules besides insulin. A human pancreas hosts several types of cells that secrete several molecules such as insulin, glucagon, somatostatin, pancreatic polypeptides, and others [14].

Therefore, there is the need to measure several molecules in order to address full monitoring of human metabolism. Moreover, if we would like to deliver and monitor several compounds, including chemotherapy and anti-inflammatory drugs, we also need to detect the best-known compounds commonly used in pharmacological treatments. Table 4.2 summarizes some of these molecules that should be targets of implantable sensors considering both endogenous (typically disease biomarkers) and exogenous (typically therapeutic drugs) molecules.

Problem of Specificity

With respect to developing IMDs able to detect all the molecules reported in Table 4.1, there is definitely a need to identify proper molecular probes that can provide specific recognition of each individual target metabolite. Antibodies are the first molecular probe that come to mind when speaking about specific recognition. Antibodies are molecules of the human immune system that have the specific function of typically recognizing exogenous molecules entering our bodies from the outside. Our immune system usually responds to the penetration of exogenous compounds by expressing specific antibodies against the foreign molecules. However, we cannot use antibodies as probe proteins if our aim is the continuous monitoring of human metabolites. The reason is that antibodies, when immobilized onto solid substrates to obtain a biosensor, become fully saturated by the target molecules after a certain amount of time due to the strong coupling between the antibodies and their antigens. Thus, no further detection is then possible with the same sensing surface. Thus, antibodies are good probes for realizing immune sensors but not IMDs.

We need to look to enzymes to obtain more reliable molecular probes capable of continuous monitoring. The reason lies in the basic working principle of enzymes. Enzymes, like all catalysts, are not reaction products. At the end of a reaction, enzymes are in exactly the same state they were in at the beginning of the reaction. A typical enzymatic reaction is that of glucose (in the form of D-glucose, abbreviated henceforth as *D-gluc*) transformed into D-gluconic acid δ-lactone (also called D-gluconic acid, or simply gluconic acid, abbreviated *D-gluc. acid*) by glucose oxidase (*GOD*). In this reaction, a special functional group of the enzyme called FAD (flavin adenine dinucleotide) acts as coenzyme, taking a hydrogen molecule from the glucose:

$$GOD/FAD + D - gluc \rightarrow GOD/FADH_2 + D - gluc.acid. \quad (1.1)$$

After the reaction, the FAD releases the acquired hydrogen molecule thanks to the presence of oxygen in the water solution:

$$GOD/FADH_2 + O_2 \rightarrow GOD/FAD + H_2O_2. \quad (1.2)$$

A hydrogen-peroxide molecule is then produced in Reaction (2). Now the GOD and its FAD are back to the initial state they were in at the beginning of Reaction (1). Thus, the GOD is now ready for another transformation of another incoming glucose molecule. Reactions (1) and (2) show that we can, in principle, use oxidases for the continuous monitoring of their substrates. Several oxidases have a specific molecule as substrate. For example, Table 4.2 reminds us that cholesterol and lactate also have a proper oxidase to help their metabolic pathways. The list of oxidase/metabolite pairs is actually longer, including oxidases for glutamate, monoamine, NADPH, lysyl, xanthine, and several other human metabolites. In all cases, the relevant oxidase may be used to develop a sensor that provides a current linearly related to the amount of the specific enzyme's substrate.

Principle of Detection with Oxidases

To realize an electrochemical sensor by following Reactions (1) and (2), we need to identify a substance that can release (or adsorb) electrons during the redox reaction [15]. That substance is hydrogen peroxide, which is one of the products in Reaction (2). Hydrogen peroxide may be oxidized by following the reaction:

$$2H_2O_2 \rightarrow O_2^+ + 2H_2O + 4e^- \quad (1.3)$$

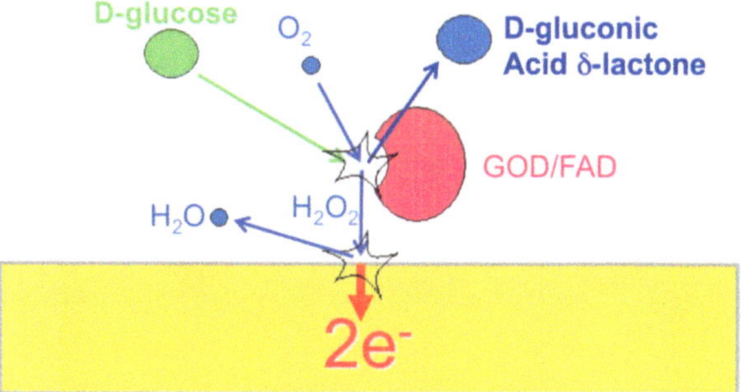

Fig. 4.3 Scheme of sensing principle involving glucose oxidase

We need to supply a potential of +650 mV to energetically support that oxidation. Therefore, we can collect the four electrons released by the hydrogen peroxide in oxidation (3) by setting a potential of +650 mV at the sensing electrode equipped with the enzymatic GOD/FAD system. Figure 4.3 schematically summarizes the basic principle of such an electrochemical sensor.

Similar reaction sequences of chain (1, 2, and 3), schematically summarized by Fig. 4.3, are possible with several other endogenous metabolites. Table 4.2 shows we can also involve cholesterol or lactate oxidase. In that case, our electrochemical sensor collects electrons always resulting from the oxidation of hydrogen peroxide at +650 mV. However, the sensor now detects the cholesterol or the lactate depending on the used oxidase.

Unfortunately, not all human metabolites have a proper oxidase that would allow for the development of a related electrochemical sensor. For example, there is no oxidase of adenosine triphosphate (ATP). Therefore, the electrochemical sensing of ATP is a bit more complex than that shown in Fig. 4.3. Table 4.2 anticipates the use of both glucose oxidase and glucose hexokinase (GHK) in that case. In fact, we need to add another reaction to chain (1, 2, and 3) to reach a specificity on ATP with an electrochemical sensor. The missing reaction involves the target ATP [16]:

$$ATP + GHK + D - gluc \rightarrow ADP + GHK + D - gluc - 6 - P. \qquad (1.4)$$

Reaction (4) shows that the GHK helps the phosphorylation of the carbon in position six of the D-glucose, giving D-glucose-6-P as byproduct. More ATP remains in the sample, less D-glucose is transformed by the GOD. The last sentence gives us the detection principle of ATP. We can realize an electrochemical sensor by mixing the glucose oxidase and the GHK. The sensor surface will consume D-glucose to produce D-glucose-6-P, while the GOD will consume D-glucose to produce H_2O_2. The consumption of D-glucose to obtain D-glucose-6-P is proportional to the amount of ATP. The remaining D-glucose is then inversely proportional to the ATP. Thus, the H_2O_2 amount, which is proportional to the remaining D-glucose, will be inversely proportional to the ATP, too.

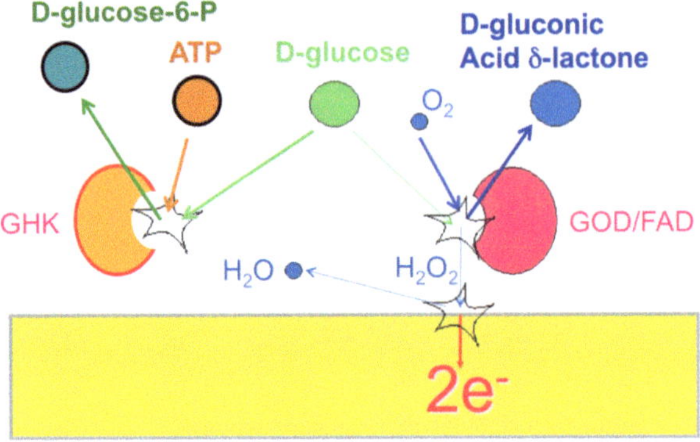

Fig. 4.4 Scheme of sensing principle involving both glucose oxidase and hexokinase

Therefore, the sensor returns a current (due to the oxidation of the H_2O_2) that is inversely proportional to the amount of ATP we have in the sample. Our electrochemical sensor is now an indirect sensor for ATP. ATP is measured with decreasing values of the registered current. As before, it is now possible to show in Fig. 4.4 the working principle of this kind of indirect electrochemical sensor, which involves both oxidases and hexokinases. We know that Reactions (1) and (2) show the possibility of continuous monitoring because the GOD/FAD is at the end of Reaction (2) in exactly the same state that it was at the beginning of Reaction (1). Analogously, Reaction (4) shows the GHK in the same state on the left as well as on the right. Thus, the GHK does not change state after Reaction (4), and therefore it can be used to transform another D-glucose molecule into D-glucose-6-P. That means this kind of sensor can assure continuous monitoring as well.

Principle of Detection of Cytochromes

Unfortunately, there are no oxidases and hexokinases for exogenous metabolites. If we want to detect an exogenous compound, we cannot develop electrochemical sensors based on oxidases. We need to look for other proteins that could be involved in electrochemical processes. We have already seen that our immune system reacts by producing specific antibodies once a foreign molecule is introduced into the body. The main aim of antibodies is to create clusters of exogenous compounds to enable phages to contrast the non-physiological compound. During evolution, nature developed another strategy: the alien compound can be oxidized in order to make it more soluble and, thus, more quickly secreted by our body. To facilitate the solubility of the exogenous compounds, evolution developed another class of enzymes: the cytochromes P450.

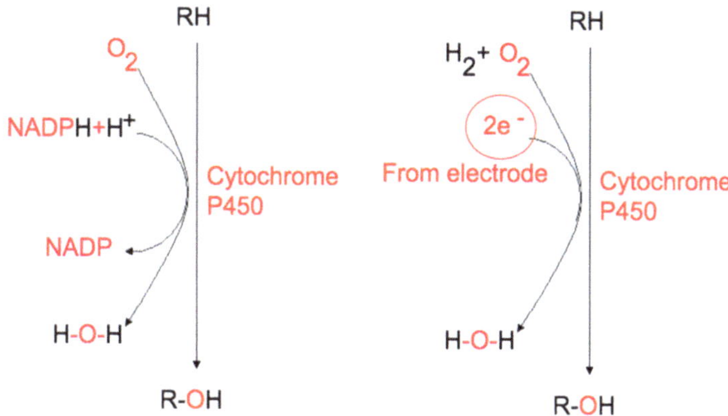

Fig. 4.5 Scheme of sensing principle involving a cytochrome P450

The cytochromes P450 is a class of proteins that participate, as catalysts, in the transformation of compounds into their oxidized forms. The typical reaction involving an enzyme of this class is in the form

$$RH + P450 + O_2 + NADPH + H^+ \rightarrow ROH + P450 + O_2 + NADP + H_2O \quad (1.5)$$

where RH is the exogenous compound, ROH its oxidized form, NADP the nicotinamide adenine dinucleotide phosphate, and NADPH its reduced form.

Reaction (5) shows again that the enzyme is unaltered after the reaction. Thus, it can be used for continuous monitoring. Moreover, Reaction (5) also shows that we can develop electrochemical sensors. In fact, looking deeper inside Reaction (5), we see that the presence of the NADPH and the proton (H^+) is due to the fact that they furnish two electrons for the reaction (Fig. 4.5). Therefore, we can detect the exogenous compound RH by just scanning the potential across the electrode interface and, thus, by furnishing the required electrons to the cytochrome in a water-based environment where the redox reaction can easily find both protons and oxygen. In that way, the scheme on the right-hand side of Fig. 4.5 shows exactly how an electrochemical sensor works based on the cytochromes P450.

Returning to Table 4.2, we see now that there are several proteins in the class of cytochromes P450 that may be used specifically to address the detection of several drugs. The table tells us that we can detect a well-known anticancer compound (cyclophosphamide) using the isoform 3A4. The commercially available anti-inflammatory compounds known as flurbiprofen and naproxen may be detected using the isoform 2C9. The isoform 2B4 detects benzphetamine. The isoform 3A4 also detects dextromethorphan (a cough suppressant).

Problem of Sensitivity

Equation 3 shows that the oxidation of hydrogen peroxide produces electrons. Collecting these electrons at the time at the interface of the sensor electrode means measuring a current. This may be done in all the reactions involving endogenous metabolites and oxidases. Thus, detection based on oxidases may occur by measuring the current generated at the electrode interface. Similarly, the scheme on the right-hand side of Fig. 4.5 indicates that the transformation of exogenous metabolites involving cytochromes requires electrons. If this reaction occurs at the surface of an electrode, then the electrode may furnish these electrons. Providing electrons upon the time at the interface of the sensor means supplying a current to the redox, and thus a measure of the current is again feasible to monitor the reaction. This is possible in all the reactions involving exogenous metabolites and cytochromes. Therefore, amperometric sensors (sensors based on current measurements) are suitable to develop IMDs for measuring all the metabolites listed in Table 4.2 and many others. The correct approach is to develop sensing electrodes based on probe enzymes similar to those listed in the left column of that table in order to specifically address the metabolites similar to those listed in the right columns of the same table. However, we could encounter a problem in developing such a sensor: the detection range supported by the sensor must fit with the physiological ranges of the metabolites in the patient's blood or in the body fluid or tissue where we plan to insert the IMD. In other words, the sensor must be sensitive enough to correctly meet the need of the application. This requirement is not trivial to address. In fact, the literature gives many examples of various sensors proposed to detect both endogenous and exogenous metabolites. All these sensors possess several features, and some of them usually define their range of operability. Among them, the most important for defining a detection range are the sensitivity, the detection limit, and the saturation level.

Let us consider the generic amperometric sensor. In general, it responds with increasing currents to increased amounts of metabolite concentration, as shown in Fig. 4.6. However, this does not happen for all the values of the target concentration.

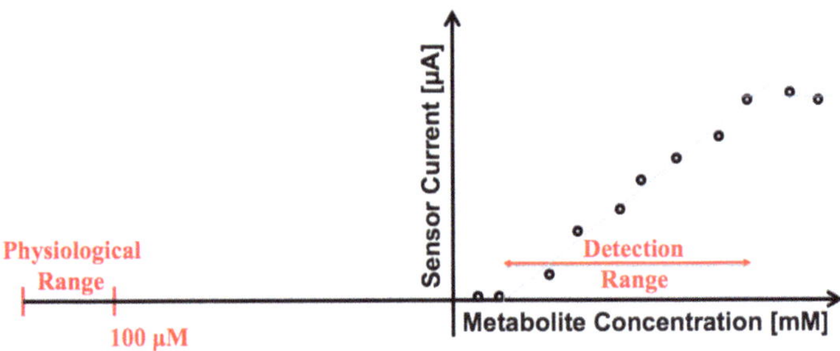

Fig. 4.6 Typical calibration curve of an electrochemical sensor compared to required physiological range of concentrations

Typically, the sensor is blind up to a certain concentration. The current measured by the sensor for concentration values smaller than that amount is typically the noise current. We call the *detection limit* the minimum value of concentration at which the sensor starts to respond with current variations significantly different from that of the noise. For values larger than the detection limit, the current registered by the sensor linearly increases with the concentration. The rate of the slope of this linear relationship between current and concentration is called the *sensitivity* of the sensor.

The sensitivity of the device defines how reliable the sensor is in detecting the target metabolite. In practice, the current stops increasing when the concentration reaches a certain maximum value. Figure 4.6 shows that the measured current increases in a linear curve (called a *calibration curve*) until a certain concentration of the metabolite is reached. For concentrations larger than a certain value, the current no longer increases. The maximum detectable concentration value is called the *saturation* of the sensor. The range of concentrations between the detection limit and the sensor saturation is called the *detection range* (Fig. 4.6). Obviously, the sensor is useful for a certain application only if its detection range fits with the physiological and physiopathological range. The two aforementioned ranges are not necessarily identical because a metabolite is typically down- or upregulated during pathology. The problem of sensitivity arises when the detection range of the sensor does not fit with the physiological or with the physiopathological range. Often, sensors proposed in the literature work very well in a certain range of concentrations. However, it happens sometimes that the physiological concentrations of the concerned metabolites are extremely low with respect to the detection limit, as schematically shown in Fig. 4.6. For example, we found in the literature sensors for ATP in the millimolar range [16] while the physiological concentration of the ATP in the interstitial tissue is in the nanomolar range [17]. Sensors for benzphetamine have been proposed in the 50 mM range [18], while the maximum concentration of benzphetamine in the blood of chronic abusers is typically below 3,000 μg/L (some patients show toxic reaction for only 20 μg/L) [19]. Verapamil has been detected with good linearity, in the millimolar range [20], while its concentration in humans is below micromoles [21]. These examples simply show that the identification of the pair metabolite/probe enzyme, as shown in Table 4.2, is not sufficient for developing metabolic sensors. The right technology also needs to provide enough sensitivity in order to succeed in developing IMDs that can actually target real medical applications.

Nanostructuring and Sensitivity Gain

There are several approaches to enhancing the performance of electrochemical sensors. Among them, the use of nanostructured electrodes has attracted considerable interest over the last 10 years. Enhanced devices have been proposed by including metallic [22] or semiconducting [23] nanoparticles, metallic nanochorals [24], carbon nanotubes (CNTs) [25, 26], carbon nanorods [27], carbon nanosheets

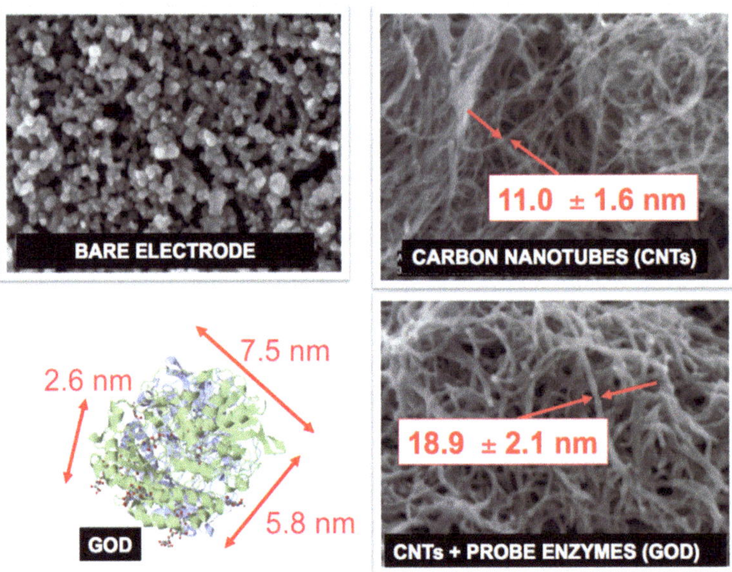

Fig. 4.7 SEM images of sensing surfaces with sizes compared with those of a glucose oxidase

(graphene) [28], and other potential nanosystems. Among these various structures, CNTs have attracted much interest due to their good performance in supporting electrical conductivity and good area/volume ratio. In recent years, we have proposed several electrochemical sensors based on CNTs for stem cell monitoring [29–31], drug detection in human serum [32, 33], and continuous monitoring of metabolic biomarkers [34, 35].

A key feature of these kinds of enhanced electrochemical sensors is to offer nanostructured networks to host the probe enzymes. Figure 4.7 gives a picture of the required structuration of an electrode surface in order to obtain such electrochemical sensors based on CNTs and enzymes. If the sensor is built starting with the commercially available screen-printed electrodes made with carbon paste, then the initial surface looks like the top-left image in Fig. 4.7 (bare electrode). This image was acquired with a scanning electron microscope (SEM) and shows the average roughness, or corrugation, of a typical screen-printed electrode realized with carbon-paste ink. The next step is the deposition of CNTs on the surface. The simplest way is to drop cast a solution of CNTs dispersed in ethanol (or chloroform) and wait a few seconds for the evaporation of the highly volatile solvent. The final result is a surface that presents features like those shown in the SEM image reported in the top right of Fig. 4.7 (CNTs). This image shows structures like tubes at the nanoscale. An average diameter of 11.0 ± 1.6 nm is registered as the average size of the fibers if the used CNTs are multiwalled structures (typically called multiwalled carbon nanotubes [MWCNT]). The next fabrication step is the deposition of the probe enzymes. The simplest way to do this is again to drop cast a water solution

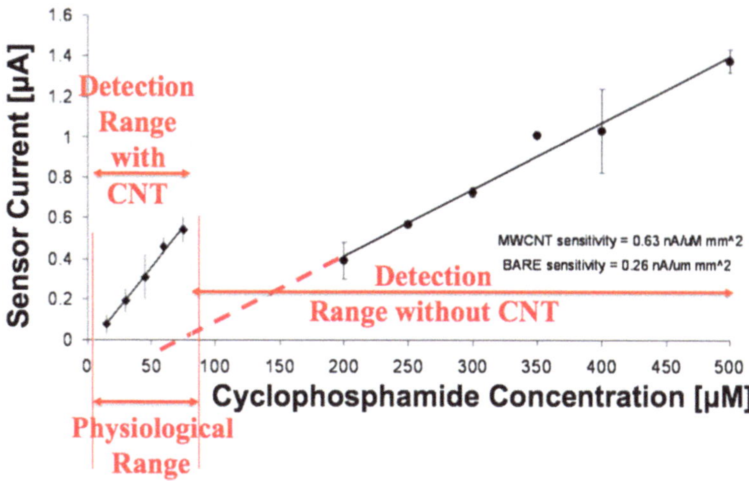

Fig. 4.8 Calibration curves of a sensor based on cytochromes P450 3A4 to sense the cyclophosphamide with and without multiwalled carbon nanotube (MWCNT)

(typically including phosphate buffered saline, also called PBS) of probe enzymes and wait a few hours for the evaporation of the water. More often, the water does not completely evaporate. However, the molecular probes are adsorbed into the CNT network in any case.

Following protein deposition with the glucose oxidase, the sensing network appears like the picture reported in the bottom right in Fig. 4.7. An average diameter of 18.9 ± 2.1 nm is registered in this SEM image as the average size of the bio/nano structuration. The structure of glucose oxidase as investigated in crystallography presents a shape like that of a parallelogram with sizes close to 6 nm (Fig. 4.7, *bottom left*) [36]. Thus, the image in Fig. 4.7 clearly indicates that just a single enzyme layer surrounds each CNT fiber. This single layer of enzymes supports the redox reactions described in Reactions (1) and (2) while the presence of CNT enhances the quantum efficiency in collecting the electrons generated in Reaction (3). Analogously, the average diameters registered in the SEM images ranges from 11.1 ± 2.6 nm before biofunctionalization to 19.5 ± 5.7 nm after biofunctionalization with cytochromes P450 3A4 [32]. The presence of several hydrophobic residues in the external surface of the cytochrome assures a strong bond energy (enthalpy) between the enzymes and the CNTs. This energy has been estimated in a range of −28 kJ/mol to −40 kJ/mol [37]. In the case of the cytochromes, the CNTs enhance the quantum efficiency in the direct electron transfer of the redox showed on the right side of Fig. 4.5.

In some cases, this kind of structuring makes a huge difference in sensing within the physiopathological or pharmacological ranges. For example, the cytochrome P450 3A4 easily detects cyclophosphamide (Table 4.2), and Fig. 4.8 clearly shows that. However, the figure shows a significant difference between sensors realized

Table 4.3 Four anticancer compounds measured with MWCNT-based sensors in both phosphate buffered saline and serum

Drug	Pharmacological range (μM)	P450 enzyme	Sensitivity (nA/μM*mm^2)		Detection limit (μM)	
			PBS	Serum	PBS	Serum
Cyclophosphamide	2.7–76.6	2B6	1.0	0.3	1.9	13.8
Ifosfamide	10–160	3A4	1.6	0.4	2.0	7.1
Ftorafur	1–10	1A2	8.8	3.5	0.7	1.0
Etoposide	34–102	–	73.7	9.1	0.1	0.5

with or without CNTs. The calibration acquired on a sensor that does not use MWCNT presents data points from 200 to 500 μM, while the concentration of cyclophosphamide found in patients' serum is below 100 μM. The sensor succeeds in obtaining data within a range of concentration from 10 up to 80 μM only when MWCNTs are used.

Thus, only the use of CNTs makes it possible to perfectly fit the pharmacological range of exogenous metabolites as found in patients' blood.

The case of P450 3A4 in detecting cyclophosphamide is not the only one. Table 4.3 summarizes other results obtained in detecting other anticancer therapeutic compounds: ifosfamide, detected again with the isoform 3A4, ftorafur with 1A2, and etoposide with MWCNT-structured electrodes without any probe enzyme [37]. Etoposide is a highly electrochemically active compound. Therefore, an enzyme is not required to enhance the redox reaction at the electrode surface. That does not happen with the other drugs given in Table 4.3. Thus, we need the right enzymes to specifically achieve detection in the other cases. All these drugs were measured in samples made using a PBS water solution and adding the drugs in a known amount. Table 4.3 shows that the detection range fits perfectly with the physiological range of the compounds. The drugs were measured in human serum, too. The serum contained all the metabolic molecules that our bodies need or produce in daily life. Therefore, the compounds were added to the commercially available serum in order to investigate the specificity of the electrochemical sensors with respect to the millions of interfering molecules in human serum.

In principle, each of these molecules could interfere with the detection of a specific compound. For example, the serum also contains glucose depending on the glycemic value of the patient. The serum also contains glucose oxidase depending on the complex metabolic control of glycemia by the patient. In principle, glucose and glucose oxidase may go through Reactions (1) and (2) and generate hydrogen peroxide, which can provide extra current to our electrochemical sensors thanks to Reaction (3). If extra currents are generated, then sensitivity can be affected. So, it is of special importance to check the sensor specificity with respect of other interfering molecules.

In the case of the anticancer compounds presented earlier, these checks were conducted [37] and the results are reported in Table 4.3. The table shows that, as expected, sensitivity goes down by a factor ranging between 88% and 61% of the value registered in the PBS. Consequently, the (DL) goes up because it is related to the sensitivity (S) by an inverse law:

$$DL = \frac{3\Delta i}{S}. \tag{1.6}$$

Equation 6 takes into account a 99.7% confidence level and explains why Table 4.3 shows an increasing detection limit on human serum. The detection limit goes up by a factor of 1.5 to 7, also depending on the noise level of the baseline (Δi). Nevertheless, the measures reported in Table 4.3 demonstrate that detection is still feasible in human serum, although the sensitivity goes down and the detection limit goes up. All the detection limits reported for serum are below the minimum amount found in patients' blood except in the case of cyclophosphamide. In this latter case, the cyclophosphamide sensor fits anyway quite well with the pharmacological range because the detection limit just slightly exceeds the minimum drug concentration found in patients. Therefore, we can conclude that all these electrochemical sensors succeed in detecting drugs in patients' blood. Similarly, the literature presents the same evidence in the case of the endogenous compounds described in Table 4.2, even if the sensitivity is still an issue in some cases. For example, it was possible to decrease the detection limit from millimolar [16] down to hundreds of micromolar [38] in the case of ATP thanks to MWCNT-based sensors. It was then possible to fit the pharmacological range when the ATP was used as the compound to treat oncologic patients [39], but the realized ATP sensor did not achieve detection in the case of the native physiological range of ATP, which is in the nanomolar range [17].

Problem of Integration

All the results mentioned earlier were obtained by drop casting solutions of CNTs and then of probe enzymes onto commercially available screen-printed working electrodes with size on the millimeter scale. In such a case, the drop casting may be easily done manually by hand-made operations. A big challenge of ongoing research in nanobioelectronics is transferring the nano- and biostructures we saw in the preceding paragraphs onto microfabricated electrodes for applications in extremely small and integrated IMDs. Several approaches are considered at present. Two of the most promising ones are microspotting and chemical vapor deposition (CVD).

The first is based on commercially available spotters that have been typically developed to deposit a few microliters of water-based solution for a microchip array [40], commonly for applications in genomics, proteomics, and metabolomics.

It is also possible to use microspotting for depositing probe enzymes (which are proteins) onto microfabricated electrochemical electrodes. The only difference is that the substrates for genomics, proteomics, and metabolomics are usually based on glass, while electrochemical electrodes are made with metals. Similarly, a mixture of

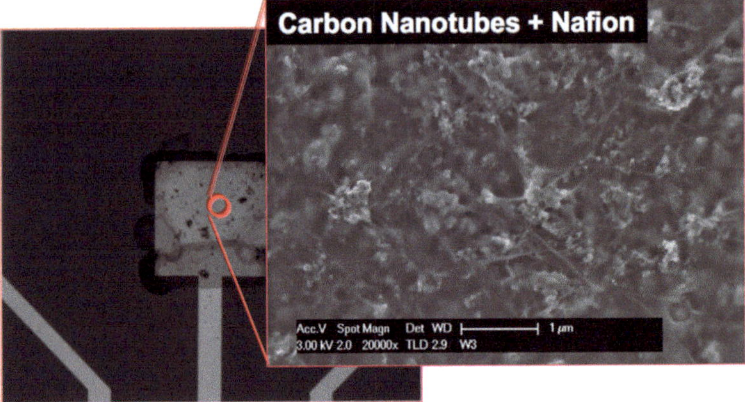

Fig. 4.9 Multiwalled carbon nanotube (MWCNT) and a polymer (Nafion) deposited onto a microelectrode using a commercially available spotter

CNTs and water-soluble polymers may be dissolved in a water solution and spread onto electrochemical microelectrodes again using microspotting. This approach was recently used to fabricate electrochemical sensors based on oxidases to realize a microsystem for continuous monitoring of cell cultures [41]. Figure 4.9 shows the results of the microspotting of CNTs. The image clearly shows that the MWCNTs are embedded in the polymer matrix, and thus the nanotube network is less dense than the case reported in Fig. 4.7. Moreover, the polymer typically surrounds the nanotube fiber, diminishing the access of the probe enzyme to the tube. As a result of this difference, the sensitivity reached with CNT microspotting is limited with respect to that obtained by direct drop casting. For example, the case of glucose detection based on glucose oxidase previously showed a limited sensitivity of only 0.46 nA mM^{-1} cm^{-2} in the case of microspotting [41], while a sensitivity of 27.7 μA mM^{-1} cm^{-2} has been obtained for the same kind of sensor realized with direct drop casting of MWCNTs dispersed on chloroform [30].

To increase the sensitivity of microfabricated electrodes for applications in IMDs, an alternative approach is to directly grow onto microchips structures made of CNTs. CVDis a technology used for growing structures by adding additional atoms dispersed in a high-pressure atmosphere directly onto substrates where catalysts are present [42]. Several types of CNTs may be directly grown onto silicon substrates using this technique (Fig. 4.10, top left).

By changing the experimental conditions, it is possible to obtain vertically staked tubes (Fig. 4.10, top right), randomly organized tubes (Fig. 4.10, bottom right), or a bent structure (Fig. 4.10, bottom left). Due to the typical symmetry of the CVD process, vertically staked structures are the easiest to obtain while randomly oriented ones are more like the structures obtained by drop casting (compare the two images in Fig. 4.10, bottomright, and Fig. 4.7, top right). However, experiments conducted to check the quantum efficiency of Reaction (3) on the structures shown in Fig. 4.9 have demonstrated that the best results are assured by bent nanotubes. In

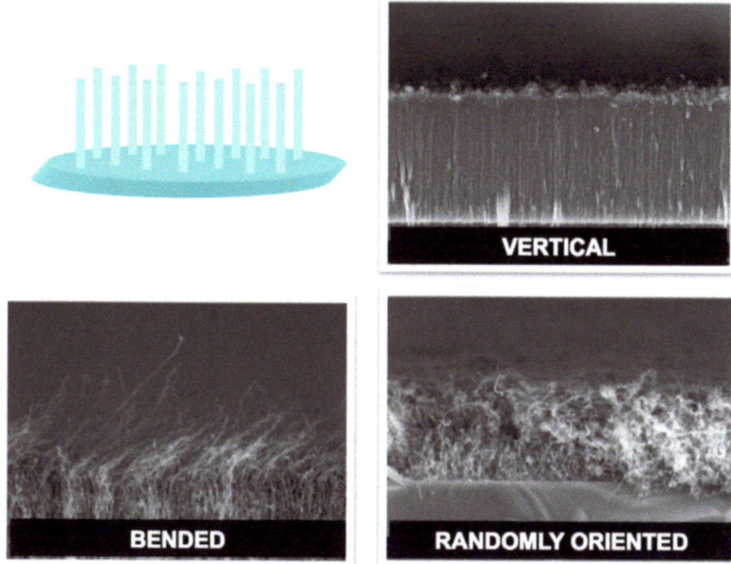

Fig. 4.10 Various kinds of carbon nanotubes directly grown on silicon substrates

fact, detection limits of 252, 1,535, and 24 μM were registered in sensing hydrogen peroxide for vertically staked, randomly oriented, and bent structures, respectively [43]. Therefore, the relative position of the tubes with respect to the substrates plays a role, too. The growth of carbon nanostructures like graphene on metallic substrates has been verified as well [44]. Therefore, it is possible to develop implantable devices by direct growth of the proper nanostructures on top of biochips to provide enhanced electrochemical detection [45].

Problem of Specificity II: The Same Enzyme for Several Substrates

Table 4.3 shows a sufficient sensitivity of electrochemical sensors based on cytochromes P450 to detect drugs in human serum. The sensor proposed with the isoform 3A4 detects cyclophosphamide in concentrations greater than 13.8 μM, which fits quite well with the expected amount in blood in a range of 2.8 to 76.6 μM. Other interfering molecules present in blood do not affect very much the detection of cyclophosphamide. However, Table 4.2 shows us that the isoform 3A4 detects dextromethorphan as well. Table 4.2 also shows that 3A4 is not the only case: the isoform 2C9 detects naproxen and flurbiprofen as well. This is a general phenomenon encountered when working with cytochromes P450 that

Table 4.4 Several substrates catalyzed by cytochromes P450 2C9

Substrate/inhibitor of CYP2C9	K_m(μM)	Ki(μM)	CYP2C9 (mV)	E_{mid} CYP2C9 + substrate (mV)
Torsemide (s)	11.4		−41	−19
Diclofenac (s)	6.8		−41	−41
Tolbutamide (s)	120		−41	−37
S-Warfarin (s)	6		−41	−36
Sulfaphenazole (i)		0.1	−41	−41
$CO_{(g)}$			−41	8

relates to the fact that these enzymes are quite different with respect to oxidases. In the case of oxidases, each enzyme has only one substrate whose redox is catalyzed by the enzyme. In the case of cytochromes P450, each enzyme instead has multiple substrates whose redox reactions are catalyzed by the same enzyme. Table 4.4 presents a very good example of the situation encountered when using these cytochromes. The table shows that the isoform 2C9 is an enzyme that catalyzes several drugs: torsemide, diclofenac, tolbutamide, s-warfarin, and sulfaphenazole [46]. It also catalyzes the redox of CO. This means we cannot hope to detect only one compound when we develop electrochemical sensors based on cytochromes P450. This is a critical problem: it seems we have insufficient specificity in pursuing the electrochemical detection of drug compounds.

Unfortunately, the solution cannot be to follow one drug at a time because patients are usually treated with drug cocktails. For example, cyclophosphamide, mitoxantrone, and etoposide are supplied together to women affected by breast cancer [47]. But not all the drug substrates of a specific P450 are supplied to patients all together. For example, torsemide is used to treat edema, diclofenac is an anti-inflammatory compound, tolbutamide is a potassium channel blocker, s-warfarin is an anticoagulant, and sulfaphenazole is an antibacterial. Thus, it is easy to think that they will not necessarily be used together. In those cases in which the compounds are present in the same therapeutic cocktail, we need to find a way to address the need to be specific enough in identifying the right exogenous compound detected by our electrochemical sensors.

We could probably try to resolve the problem by distinguishing between the different drugs contributions using a kind of voltage spectroscopy. In fact, Table 4.4 shows that the redox peak of an enzyme (indicated with the acronym CYP2C9 in the table) is located at −41 mV when there are no specific substrates in the solution. The peak remains located at −41 mV when the enzyme catalyzes diclofenac or sulfaphenazole. However, the peak shifts to −19 mV in the case of torsemide, to −37 mV with tolbutamide, and to −36 mV in the case of s-warfarin. Thus, diclofenac and sulfaphenazole are not distinguishable at all. It is hard to distinguish tolbutamide and s-warfarin because the difference in the peak locations is only 1 mV. However, it is feasible to distinguish torsemide and diclofenac because their peaks are located at a sufficient distance on the millivolt scale.

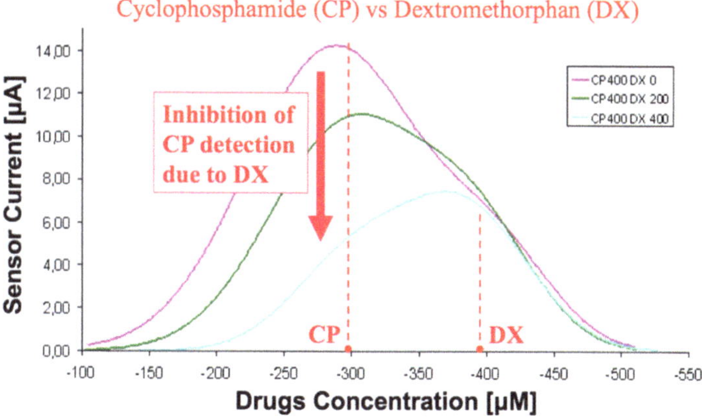

Fig. 4.11 Simultaneous detection of cyclophosphamide and dextromethorphan

Let us consider two cases of drug compounds that may be used in combination. We have already seen that cyclophosphamide is an anticancer drug. Dextromethorphan is an anticough drug.

Table 4.2 shows that both are detectable by the enzyme 3A4. An oncological patient with a cough should be treated for the cough as well. Thus, such a patient would have both drugs circulating in his or her blood. If an electrochemical sensor is developed with the isoform 3A4, then the sensor would detect both drugs [32], as shown in Fig. 4.11. This figure clearly shows a double peak in the current registered, with the voltage ranging from −100 to −550 mV. However, the two peaks are located at distinctly different positions in voltage, one at −296 mV, the other at −392 mV. A difference of almost 100 mV is easily detected, and therefore the two drugs may be uniquely identified. Another similar example is that related to well-known anti-inflammatory compounds, naproxen and flurbiprofen [32]. Because both are anti-inflammatory compounds, it is typical to find them associated in the same therapy. Table 4.2 indicates that these two compounds are also detectable using the same enzyme, the isoform 2C9. Thus, an electrochemical sensor can be developed based on this enzyme and simultaneous detection attempted. Figure 4.11 shows simultaneous detection by, again, two well-distinguished peaks.

Here, the peak of flurbiprofen is very close to −50 mV, while that of naproxen is close to 0 mV. The distance between the peaks is again quite large, and therefore we can easily identify the two drugs before quantifying their levels by the current value of the peaks.

However, once the two compounds have been correctly identified, the exact quantification of their amount is by no means trivial. In fact, both Figs. 4.10 and 4.11 show that the maximal current reached by each peak in both figures is not only related to the concentration of a single drug. In cyclic voltammetry (e.g., the acquisition of redox current by a sweep in voltage across the right potentials) the faradaic peak is usually directly proportional to the concentration of the redox compound (Randle-Sevčik equation) [15]:

$$I_{peak} \propto nFAD\sqrt{\frac{nF\nu D}{RT}}[C], \tag{1.7}$$

where F is the Faraday constant, D the diffusion coefficient of the detected redox species (the metabolite), n the number of electrons involved in the redox reaction, A the electrode area, R the Boltzmann constant, ν the voltage scan velocity, and $[C]$ the concentration of the redox species. Equation 7 indicates that the peak height is directly proportional to the metabolite concentration. By subtracting the baseline (typically related to capacitive phenomena at the interface [15]), we can describe (in a first approximation) the current acquired during the voltammetric scan by a series of Gaussian peaks:

$$i(V) = \sum_{\forall k} I_k e^{-\frac{(V-V_k)^2}{\sigma_k}}, \tag{1.8}$$

where $\boldsymbol{I_k}$ is calculated by Eq. 7, $\boldsymbol{Vk}$ is the peak position in voltage, and $\boldsymbol{\sigma_k}$ is the peak width.

However, Fig. 4.11 clearly shows that the Faradaic current of cyclophosphamide is depressed by increasing amounts of dextromethorphan. Similarly, but with the opposite result, Fig. 4.11 shows that the Faradaic current of flurbiprofen is clearly enhanced by increasing amounts of naproxen. In both experiments, only one drug's concentration is changed, while flurbiprofen and cyclophosphamide show different heights of peak currents for exactly the same value of their respective concentrations. This fact clearly indicates that Eq. 8 is no longer valid in those cases. The Faradaic currents are related to the compound providing the peak and to the level of other interfering drugs in the sample. To take into account such a complex scenario, the following equation was recently proposed [32]:

$$i(V) = \sum_{\forall k} I_k \prod_{\forall j \neq k} A_k(C_j)\, e^{-\frac{(V-V_k)^2}{\sigma_k}}. \tag{1.9}$$

In this new equation, we can clearly see that the term describing each single Gaussian component is also driven by the concentration of the other interfering drugs. The product of the different $\boldsymbol{A_k(C_j)}$ take into account these interactions. Figures 4.11 and 4.12 show examples of two different kinds of interference: inhibition and activation. Figure 4.12 shows that increasing amounts of naproxen activate the detection of flurbiprofen, while Fig. 4.11 shows that increasing amounts of dextromethorphan inhibit the detection of cyclophosphamide. These two cases correspond to different $\boldsymbol{A_k(C_j)}$ terms.

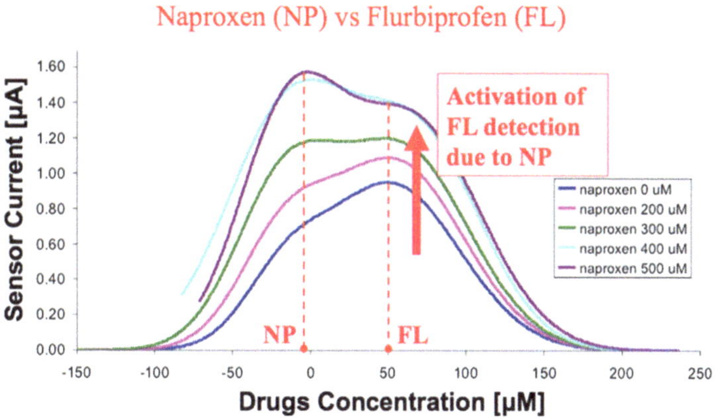

Naproxen (NP) vs Flurbiprofen (FL)

Activation of FL detection due to NP

naproxen 0 uM
naproxen 200 uM
naproxen 300 uM
naproxen 400 uM
naproxen 500 uM

Sensor Current [μA]

Drugs Concentration [μM]

NP

FL

Fig. 4.12 Simultaneous detection of naproxen and flurbiprofen

In the case of activation, we can write [32]

$$A_k(C_j) = A_{k0}\left(1 + \varepsilon_j \frac{V_{MAX}C_j}{K_M + C_j}\right) \tag{1.10}$$

while in the case of inhibition, we can write [32]

$$A_k(C_j) = A_{k0}\left(1 - \varepsilon_j \frac{V_{MAX}C_j}{K_M + C_j}\right). \tag{1.11}$$

Equations 9 and 10 describe the case of naproxen and flurbiprofen, shown in Fig. 4.12, while Eqs. 9 and 11 describe the case of dextromethorphan and cyclophosphamide, shown in Fig. 4.11. In both Eqs. 10 and 11, the term involving V_{MAX} and K_M corresponds to the Michaelis-Menten kinetics usually considered for all enzymes, while the term ε_j takes into account the strength of the interaction. In some cases, the cytochromes P450 follow atypical kinetics, which are different than the Michaelis-Menten kinetics. Of course, an exhaustive discussion on the atypical kinetics of P450s and on the causes of the different kinds of interactions of their substrates is outside the scope of this book. For a more detailed discussion, interested readers may refer to Chap. 4 in Ref. [15].

Equations 10 and 11 are nonlinear equations with respect to the concentration of the interfering drugs. The Michaelis-Menten term returns a double dependence on C_j of A_k. Therefore, a linear approach to an automatic decoupling of the different drug contributions is not possible. However, there are some concentration ranges in which a simpler linear approach is still possible. Let us consider once again the case of the drugs in Table 4.3. Imagine a multipanel platform having on board four electrochemical sensors developed with the P450 enzymes listed in the table. If we consider several protocols usually used to treat oncology patients with breast cancer [47–50], we can easily see that cyclophosphamide, ftorafur, and ifosfamide are never

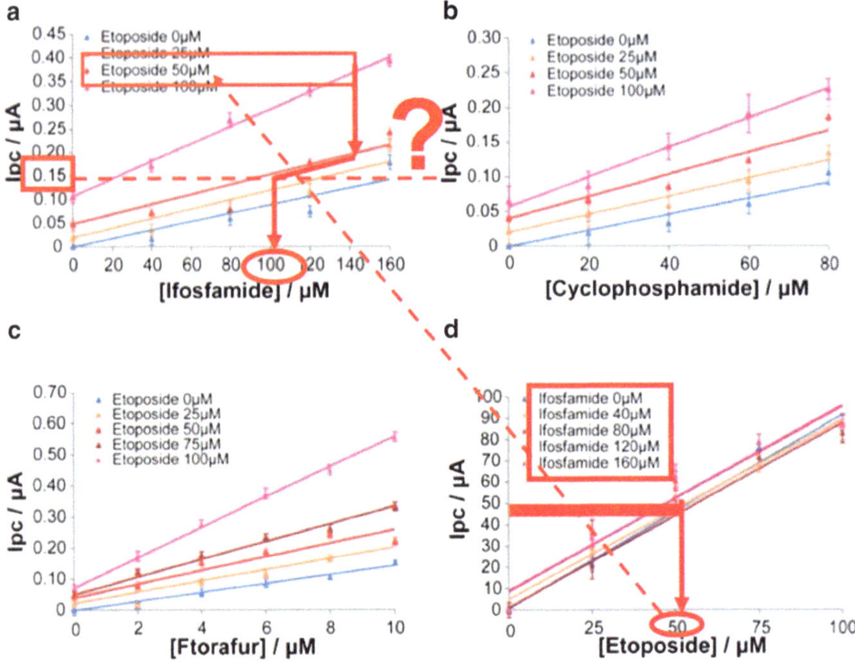

Fig. 4.13 Families of calibration curves acquired with the P450-based sensors described by Table 4.3

used together, but etoposide is always used together with the others. Thus, we face a situation like that shown in Fig. 4.13 using a platform based on Table 4.3. The presence of etoposide always changes the current corresponding to the detection of cyclophosphamide, ftorafur, and ifosfamide. The same thing probably does not happen on the sensor measuring etoposide. Graph D in the bottom right of Fig. 4.13 shows that the interaction of ifosfamide with the detection of etoposide is within the range experimental error. Thus, ifosfamide does not interfere with the detection of etoposide. Similar graphs have been produced in the case of cyclophosphamide and ftorafur.

Therefore, we can use the information we collect at the system level with our platform to decouple the contributions of all the simultaneously detected drugs. Let us consider now one example. If we detect 0.15 µA of current with a sensor hosting the isoform 3A4, then we cannot calculate the concentration of ifosfamide because we do not know which calibration curve we need to consider. To properly navigate all the calibration curves in graph A of Fig. 4.13, we need to know the concentration of etoposide. We will likely be able to read the current registered by sensor D (assume 45 µA) and deduce the amount of etoposide in the sample (50 µM). Returning now to sensor A, we can correctly identify the correct calibration curve (that for 50 µM of etoposide), and therefore we can correctly estimate the amount of ifosfamide in our sample (100 µM in our example).

This simple example shows that we can manage to correctly distinguish each drug contribution if we operate at the system level. However, the three graphs A–C of Fig. 4.13 remind us that the drug–drug interactions are not linear. For example, the calibration curve on ftorafur in graph C presents a steeper slope for 100 μM of etoposide than for only 25 μM. The same observation may be made in comparing the different calibration curves of cyclophosphamide and ftorafur in graphs A and B. Nevertheless, the detection of all these three drugs is linearly affected by etoposide in a range of 0–50 μM. Therefore, a linear approach is possible in that range of concentrations. Thus, in a first approximation, we can also write that [51]

$$c = S^{-1} i \tag{1.12}$$

in matrix form, where $S \in R^{nxm}$ is the matrix of sensitivities, i the column matrix of currents of all the sensors, and c the raw matrix of all the drug concentrations. In Eq. 12, each s_{ij} component of matrix S is the current returned by sensor i on drug j, and the equation gives the concentrations of all the drugs in case S is fully invertible. The approach proposed by Eq. 12 is not always valid, as shown by Eqs. 10 and 11, but it may be very useful in developing biochips for identifying and quantifying drugs in patient tissues for applications in fully automatic IMDs.

Design of Smart Multiplexed Platforms

Equation 7 says that we can estimate the concentration of a metabolite by measuring a current. Figures 4.11 and 4.12 show that a reliable detection of multiple drugs is possible only by a voltage scan. Equation 12 tells us that a data processor is required in any case to correctly quantify the metabolites. Tables 4.2 and 4.3 indicate that we need multipanel platforms in order to develop IMDs that measure several metabolites related to human metabolism. Table 4.3 and Fig. 4.13 show enzymes that especially need to work at the system level in order to be specific enough in detection. Table 4.2 shows that detection is simpler in the case of endogenous metabolites because oxidases are more specific enzymes. However, even endogenous metabolites require a system-level approach to improve specificity, as in the case of ATP whose detection depends on the amount of glucose (Eq. 4 and Fig. 4.4).

In the face of all this complexity, we need to address the development of very smart multiplexed platforms to provide fully telemetry of human metabolism. A general architecture that was proposed recently is presented in Fig. 4.14 [52]. This architecture shows that a data processing unit is the core at the system level. It can generate fixed (for oxidase-based sensors) or variable (for P450-based sensors) potentials. These voltages are correctly applied to the microfabricated sensors of the chip. This requires a potentiostat on board. From each sensor the chip needs to measure the currents collected by the sensing electrodes. This means that we also need to have on board a multiplexer that properly manages all these

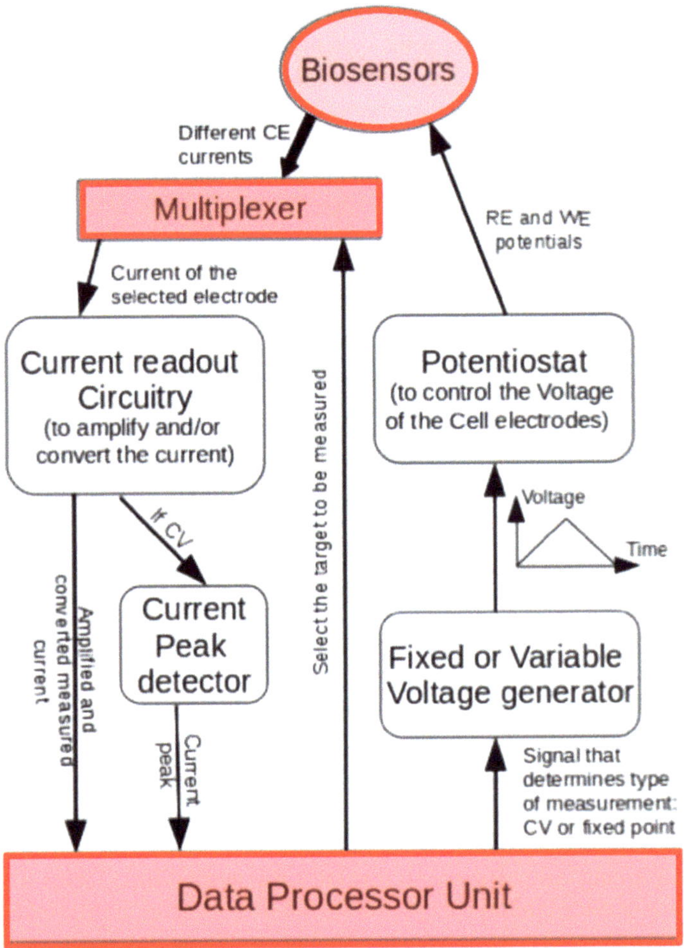

Fig. 4.14 Possible block scheme of a multipanel IMD

sensors. A current readout circuit amplifies and converts the measured current into more reliable signals (typically a voltage or a frequency). Finally, a peak detector estimates the metabolite concentration.

A detailed description of processing units, analog multiplexers, and potentiostats is beyond the scope of this book. The interested reader may refer to Chap. 13 in Ref. [53], which presents a very basic and clear description of how to design a simple CMOS potentiostat. Current readout circuits that amplify and convert currents into more reliable signals (typically a voltage [53] or a frequency [54]) are reported in the literature as well. Readers may also consult Chap. 3 of Ref. [55] for a basic introduction to processing units. Analog multiplexers are presented in Chap. 3 of Ref. [56].

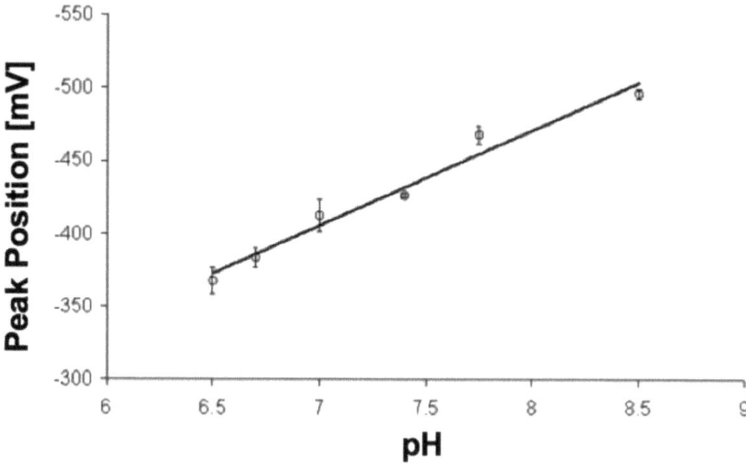

Fig. 4.15 Peak position dependence on pH of a P450-based sensor

Instead, this chapter focuses on certain specific problems that are usually not addressed in the literature but are in fact encountered in developing IMDs for real applications. We now turn to three specific problems: the reliability of pH and temperature in human tissue and the fully onboard generation of the required voltage ramps.

With regard to pH, we need to consider that the peak positions discussed earlier are given by the full Nernst equation [15]:

$$V_k = V_0 + \frac{RT}{nF} \ln \left[\frac{C_o}{C_R} \right] - \frac{RT}{nF} pH, \tag{1.13}$$

where *R, T, F, n* are the same as in Eq. 7, V_k is the peak position in Eqs. 8 and 9, and V_0 is called a standard potential. Equation 13 shows that the presence of hydrogen ions directly changes the peak location in an inverse linear relation. Figure 4.15 shows the degree to which the pH contribution in Eq. 13 affects the peak location in P450-based detection. The figure clearly shows that a slight variation of only one point of pH around the physiological value results in a peak shift of approximately 80 mV [57]. This value is close to the difference in the peak location of dextromethorphan and cyclophosphamide in Fig. 4.10, which is slightly less than 100 mV. It is also close to the peak location difference of slightly more than 50 mV in the case of naproxen and Flurbiprofen. Table 4.4 shows that the peaks of tolbutamide and s-warfarin are located at a distance of only 1 mV from each other.

Therefore, a very precise estimation of the pH is required to correctly identify the peak locations so as to correctly identify the metabolites. Even in the case of redox involving oxidases we are operating under the law of Eq. 13. Thus, even in that case, an incorrect control of the pH results in an incorrect estimation of the metabolites because the current is changing due to a progressive shift of the redox energy. Thus,

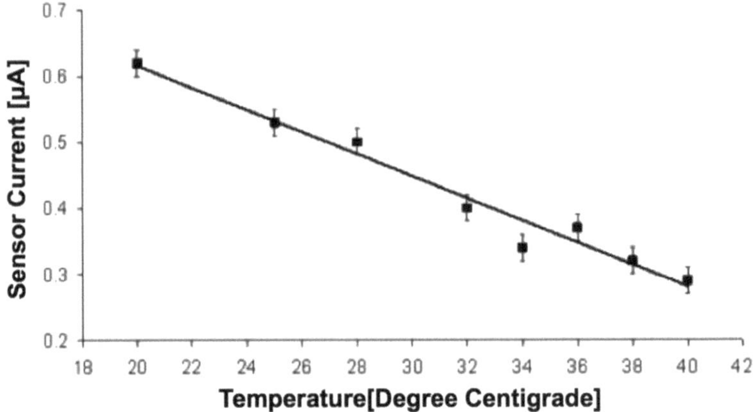

Fig. 4.16 Peak current dependence on T of a P450-based sensor

in the cases of both endogenous and exogenous metabolites, a precise measure of the pH is strictly required in order to correctly calibrate the identification and the estimation of the metabolic compounds in human tissues.

Similarly, we need to calibrate for temperature (T). In fact, both Eqs. 7 and 13 depend on temperature. A change in body temperature results in a change in both the position and maximum current of the redox peak. Figure 4.16 shows that the current changes from 0.4 to 0.3 μA in the case of a patient with fever. That means an error of approximately 25% in the estimation of the metabolite concentration if we do not measure and calibrate for temperature variations.

Therefore, a precise measure of the temperature is also required in order to correctly calibrate the estimation of the metabolic compounds in human tissues.

Another important issue is the onboard full generation of ramps. We need subhertz voltage ramps to address the acquisition of signals like those reported in Figs. 4.11 and 4.12. There are several examples in the literature of voltage generation on a chip. However, almost all the proposed cases are in megahertz [58] or gigahertz [60] frequency ranges, though several cases are reported of subhertz ranges, and in most of these, the ramp is not fully generated on board. The reason is that ramps are usually generated using RC circuits, as shown in the scheme of Fig. 4.17 (top left). In those cases, the capacitance or current required values are usually not compatible with integrated circuits (ICs) that are a few millimeters in size. Of course, we also need to consider minimally invasive devices when developing fully implantable IMDs for human telemetry. That means we need to have biochips with areas of a few millimeters, and therefore, capacitors of hundreds of microfarad and currents of picoampere cannot be considered.

We need new approaches to obtaining ramps generated fully on board. A mixed-signal solution was recently proposed to resolve the problem [59]. As shown in Fig. 4.17 (bottom right), the proposed architecture foresees a reference oscillator that is used to drive an addition/subtraction unit that charges an accumulator. The

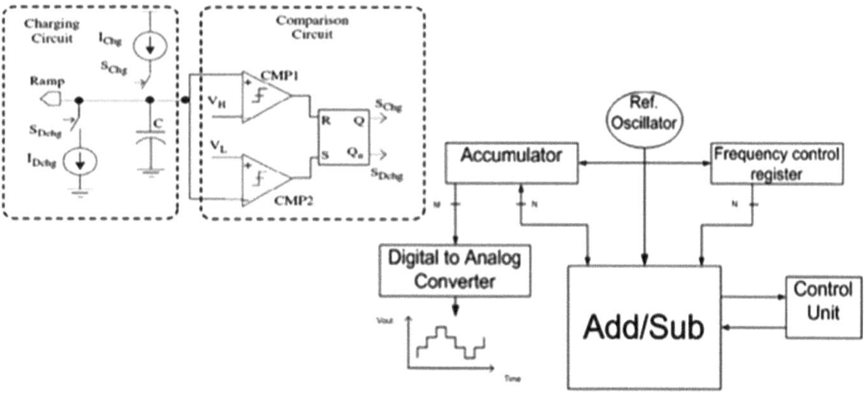

Fig. 4.17 Two methods for voltage ramp generation

accumulator presents as output a time-series of numbers that are then converted into a digitized increasing or decreasing ramp by a digital-to-analog converter. In this manner, voltage ramps with the proper voltage-scanning rate (in a range of 10 mV/s) have been successfully generated with an IC of only 1.5 × 1.5 mm [61].

Realizing Smart Remotely Powered Platforms

The innovative multipanel platforms discussed in the preceding sections could be used to realize extremely integrated and remotely powered IMDs as new tools in personalized medicine. One idea investigated and proposed recently in the literature is that of an extremely small multisensor to be fully located in the interstitial tissue under the skin [35]. To assure minimal sizes in implants, the device cannot host batteries. Therefore, the IMD requires remote powering by an electronic patch located on top of the skin (Fig. 4.18) [62].

The patch transmits power to the IMD and receives data from the IMD. The patch retransmits the acquired data to a smartphone or a tablet. The core of the system is the IMD, which is of a novel conception. It hosts (Fig. 4.19) up to five different molecular sensors, one sensor to measure the local temperature, one sensor to measure the local pH, a dedicated IC, and a smart antenna built in three dimensions in order to fit inside small devices. The idea was to develop an IMD that might have the sizes of a large surgery needle in order to be minimally invasive. The five molecular sensors can measure different metabolites depending on the probe enzymes immobilized on the sensing electrodes. The temperature and pH sensors are required to calibrate the currents (Fig. 4.16) and their peak locations (Fig. 4.15) registered by the molecular sensors.

The dedicated IC [61, 63] is the sensors frontend circuit required by all the onboard sensors as well as the circuit necessary to rectify the received power signal.

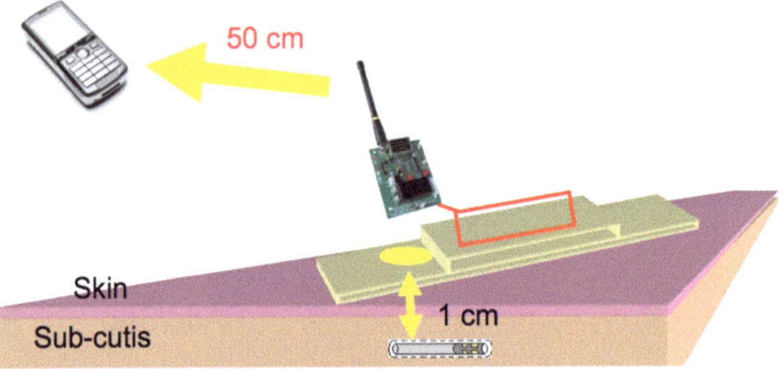

Fig. 4.18 A system for personalized medicine composed of an IMD located under the skin, a patch located on top of the skin, and a smartphone

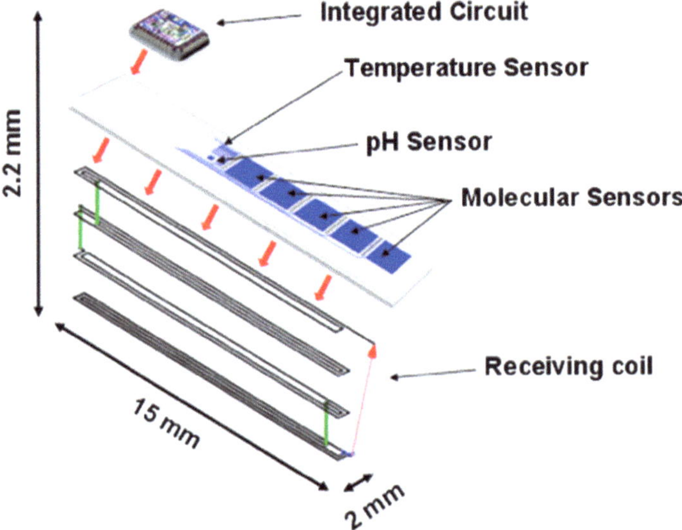

Fig. 4.19 A remotely powered IMD the size of a large surgery needle

This signal is provided by an inductive link that operates at less than 5 MHz [64]. It has been demonstrated that 2 GHz is required to optimize the power transmission for transmitting and receiving coils that are both on the millimeter scale [65], while the optimal frequency is scaled down to the megahertz range when only the receiving coil is on the millimeter scale and the transmitting one remains on the centimeter scale [66]. The received power is unavoidably extremely low (below 1%) if the receiving antenna needs to remain limited by very few millimeters. A link efficiency of 1% is too low both in terms of the required huge amount of transmitted energy and in terms of the power dissipation in human tissue.

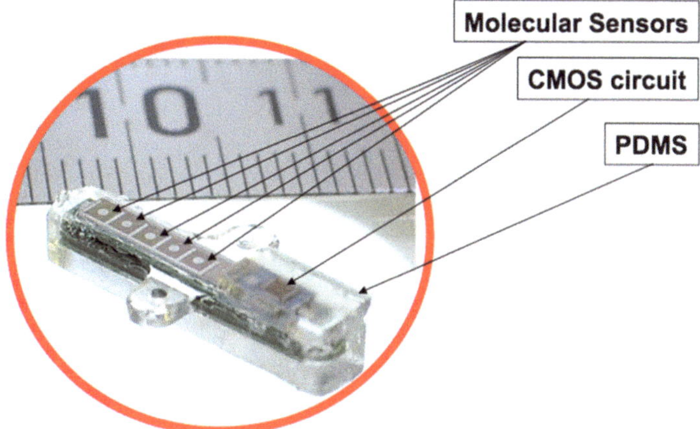

Fig. 4.20 Innovative IMD including biocompatible PDMS packaging

To solve this problem, a multilayer spiral inductor was developed in the z-direction (Fig. 4.18). An efficiency of up to 25% for the inductive link was then obtained with the two coils positioned 6 mm each other using this antenna [64]. Experiments conducted with a transmitting planar coil up to 24×38 mm in size and a multilayer spiral inductor as small as 0.9×38 mm (single turn) returned a transferred power of 1.17 mW [64], while a power of only 80 μW (with 1.8 V supply voltage) is frontend sensor fabricated using in 0.18 μm UMC technology in the case of a lactate measure [63]. Therefore, the feasibility of a remotely powered IMD for multipanel detection of several metabolites has been demonstrated. Such an IMD was effectively built by integrating the multilayer spiral inductor, the fabricated IC, a passive silicon platform that hosts the seven sensors, and biocompatible silicon packaging in order to assure the required biocompatibility (Fig. 4.20). This development was effectively accomplished taking into account the very small size envisioned for minimally invasive applications, as illustrated by Fig. 4.21. The device is currently under testing with animal models to verify biocompatibility as well as working functions.

The Problem of Security

In human telemetry, another very important issue has to be considered: the security involved in working with implanted devices. In principle, we need to provide reliable and secure behavior once a biochip is implanted in a patient's body. We need to be sure that the system is always working properly, especially if the implanted device involves a kind of surveillance on the patient. We need to avoid situations in which an alarm is generated because the reproducibility of the sensors is faulty

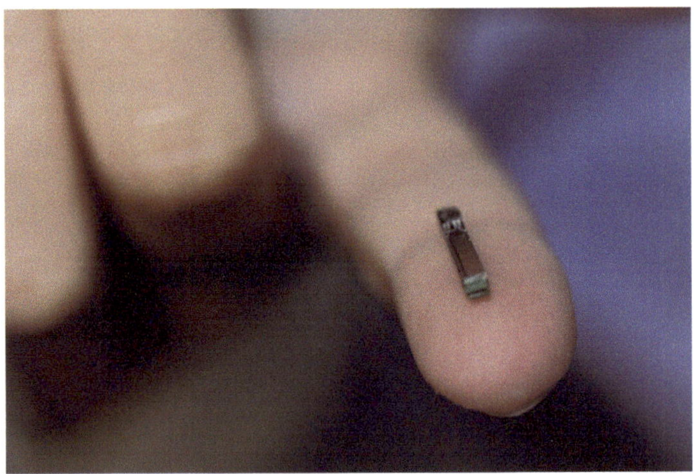

Fig. 4.21 Comparison of sizes between IMD and a human finger

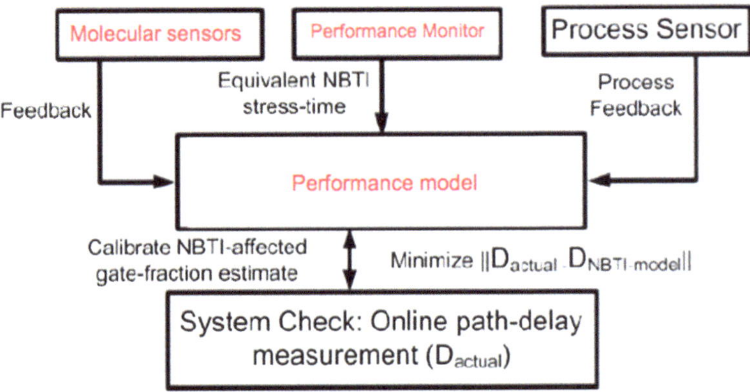

Fig. 4.22 Proposed architecture to check on sensor reproducibility

and not because a disease biomarker (a metabolite related to the patient's disease) is entering a dangerous range.

A good approach to resolving this issue was recently published [67]. Although the proposed model has been demonstrated for a temperature sensor, it is easily extendible to the more complex biosensing platforms discussed in this chapter. The proposed approach uses a performance model (Fig. 4.22) to control the behavior of the sensors on board. The behavior of the sensors is monitored on the basis of the performance model previously implemented in the system. The security-check system then tries to minimize the difference between the actual measure and the measure value expected with respect to the implemented performance model. Once the security system has repeated several minimization trials, the data are transmitted, with a certain probability that they are accurate. With this approach, the reliability of the sensors is further improved and the risk of erroneous data generation is minimized.

The Problem of Privacy

When dealing with IMDs, we also need to provide security as well as privacy in communicating the data collected by the implants to the telemedicine cloud. An approach to improving privacy in medical data communication was recently proposed [68]. This approach takes into account that several links must be protected when dealing with IMDs implanted in the body of a patient (Fig. 4.23).

Figure 4.23 shows that a patient's personal data acquisition (PDA) system is the first link in more close proximity to the implants. In Fig. 4.23, the PDA is the mobile phone of the patient. In other cases (e.g., GlucoMen Day by A. Menarini Diagnostics described in Chap. 2 [6]), it may be a point-of-care download system carried by nurses or doctors. In all cases, this is the first link in which we might experience a hostile attack from nonauthorized persons attempting to access the implant. To diminish the risk of data intrusions, a certificate authority (CA) is delegated to authorize full access to the data stored in the memory located near the sensory devices. This can be easily accomplished to authorize data access with devices located closer to the patient and his IMDs. However, this is not enough for remote communication from a PDA device or from implanted devices directly to the hospital or to the telecare center that is constantly monitoring the patient. In this case, data encryption would be required to guarantee safe remote data transmission.

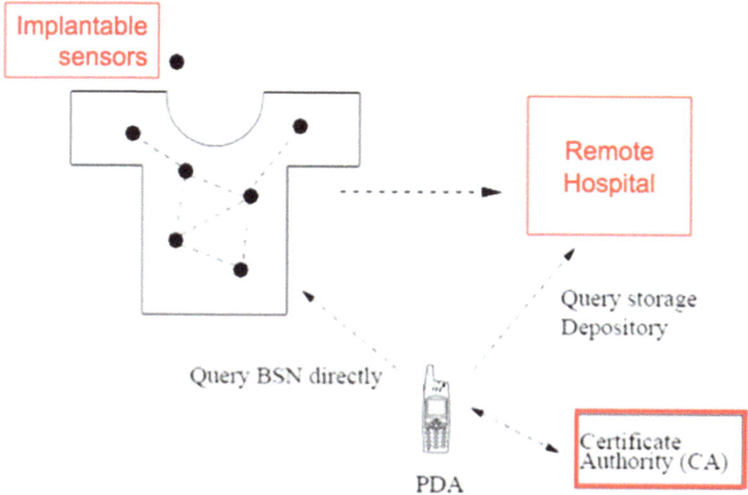

Fig. 4.23 Several links involved in connecting IMDs with a remote hospital

Conclusions

This chapter focused on specific solutions for designing innovative and smart IMDs. We saw the feasibility of developing new systems for the telemetry of human metabolism. Multisensor platforms are required to bring this about. Such platforms could be based on electrochemical sensors that host the proper enzymes to address specific detection of both endogenous and exogenous metabolites. In the same cases, specificity is not completely assured by the enzyme/metabolite pair, and therefore further strategies at the system level must be implemented in order to improve the specificity of the whole system. Sensitivity is often not assured by simply functionalizing the sensor electrodes with the right enzymes. Often, nanostructures such as CNTs are required in order to reach the right detection limit for sensing the metabolites at the right concentrations in human tissue. Assuring calibrated measures with fully implanted IMDs also requires implementing pH and temperature control as well as special mixed-signal architectures for generating the right signals. Once the implants are developed, issues of security and privacy need to be taken into account. Thus, the chapter also briefly mentioned recently proposed approaches to addressing security and privacy issues. However, the aim of the first part of this book is mainly focused on sensing technology. Therefore, readers are urged to consult Chaps. 6 and 7 of the book for a deeper discussion and more details regarding the security and privacy of IMDs.

Acknowledgments I must acknowledge several people for the ideas and scientific results contained in this chapter. First of all, I would like to thank Nanni (Giovanni De Micheli) for his contribution to and continuous support of my research. I must also thank all my Ph.D. students who have toiled in the lab over the years. In particular, I must thank Cristina Boero for Figs. 4.7 and 4.9; Irene Taurino for Fig. 4.10; Andrea Cavallini, who acquired and elaborated all the results reported in Figs. 4.8, 4.11, and 4.12; Camilla Baj-Rossi, who worked hard to acquire all the data necessary to define the calibration-curve families reported in Fig. 4.13 and to develop the linear approach proposed by Eq. 12; Sara Seyedeh Ghoreishizadeh, who designed, realized, and tested the systems in Figs. 4.14 and 4.17; and Jacopo Olivo, who drew Fig. 4.19. I also thank Roland Thewes, from the Technical University of Berlin, for providing me with Fig. 4.2. Finally, special thanks go to Wayne Burleson, who shed light for me on issues related to security and privacy in implantable medical devices.

References

1. B. B. Spear, M. Heath-Chiozzi, and J. Huff, "Clinical application of pharmacogenetics," *Trends in Molecular Medicine,* vol. 7, pp. 201–204, 5/1/2001.
2. P. B. H. C. P. N. Lazarou J, "Incidence of adverse drug reactions in hospitalized patients: A meta-analysis of prospective studies," *JAMA,* vol. 279, pp. 1200–1205, 1998.
3. J. de Leon, M. T. Susce, and E. Murray-Carmichael, "The AmpliChip™ CYP450 Genotyping Test," *Molecular diagnosis & therapy,* vol. 10, pp. 135–151, 2006.
4. K. Jain, "Personalized medicine," *Current opinion in molecular therapeutics,* vol. 4, p. 548, 2002.

5. L. C. Clark, Jr., Wolf, R, Granger, D, and Taylor, Z. :, , "Continuous recording of blood oxygen tension by polarography," *J. Appi. Physiol.*, vol. 6, pp. 189–193, 1953.
6. F. Valgimigli, F. Lucarelli, C. Scuffi, S. Morandi, and I. Sposato, "Evaluating the clinical accuracy of GlucoMen® Day: a novel microdialysis-based continuous glucose monitor," *Journal of diabetes science and technology,* vol. 4, p. 1182, 2010.
7. P. Cong, N. Chaimanonart, W. H. Ko, and D. J. Young, "A wireless and batteryless 10-bit implantable blood pressure sensing microsystem with adaptive RF powering for real-time laboratory mice monitoring," *Solid-State Circuits, IEEE Journal of,* vol. 44, pp. 3631–3644, 2009.
8. L. Bolomey, E. Meurville, and P. Ryser, "Implantable ultra-low power DSP-based system for a miniature chemico-rheological biosensor," *Procedia Chemistry,* vol. 1, pp. 1235–1238, 2009.
9. A. Poscia, D. Messeri, D. Moscone, F. Ricci, and F. Valgimigli, "A novel continuous subcutaneous lactate monitoring system," *Biosensors and bioelectronics,* vol. 20, pp. 2244–2250, 2005.
10. T. Tan, S. W. Watts, and R. P. Davis, "Drug delivery: enabling technology for drug discovery and development. iPRECIO® Micro Infusion Pump: programmable, refillable, and implantable," *Frontiers in pharmacology,* vol. 2, 2011.
11. R. M. Bergenstal, W. V. Tamborlane, A. Ahmann, J. B. Buse, G. Dailey, S. N. Davis, *et al.*, "Effectiveness of sensor-augmented insulin-pump therapy in type 1 diabetes," *New England Journal of Medicine,* vol. 363, pp. 311–320, 2010.
12. R. A. P. De Carvalho, A. L. Murphree, and E. E. Schmitt, "Implantable and sealable medical device for unidirectional delivery of therapeutic agents to tissues," ed: Google Patents, 2010.
13. G. Steil, A. Panteleon, and K. Rebrin, "Closed-loop insulin delivery—the path to physiological glucose control," *Advanced drug delivery reviews,* vol. 56, pp. 125–144, 2004.
14. H.-G. Beger, M. Buchler, R. Kozarek, M. Lerch, J. Neoptolemos, A. Warshaw, *et al.*, *The pancreas: an integrated textbook of basic science, medicine, and surgery*: Wiley-Blackwell, 2009.
15. S. Carrara, *Bio/CMOS interfaces and co-design*: Springer, 2012.
16. F. Scheller and D. Pfeiffer, "Glucose oxidase—hexokinase bienzyme electrode sensor for adenosine triphosphate," *Analytica Chimica Acta,* vol. 117, pp. 383–386, 1980.
17. U. Schenk, M. Frascoli, M. Proietti, R. Geffers, E. Traggiai, J. Buer, *et al.*, "ATP inhibits the generation and function of regulatory T cells through the activation of purinergic P2X receptors," *Science signaling,* vol. 4, p. ra12, 2011.
18. V. Shumyantseva, T. Bulko, Y. O. Rudakov, G. Kuznetsova, N. Samenkova, A. Lisitsa, *et al.*, "Electrochemical properties of cytochroms P450 using nanostructured electrodes: direct electron transfer and electro catalysis," *Journal of inorganic biochemistry,* vol. 101, p. 859, 2007.
19. C. Engblom, T. Gunnar, A. Rantanen, and P. Lillsunde, "Driving under the influence of drugs-amphetamine concentrations in oral fluid and whole blood samples," *Journal of analytical toxicology,* vol. 31, pp. 276–280, 2007.
20. S. Joseph, J. F. Rusling, Y. M. Lvov, T. Friedberg, and U. Fuhr, "An amperometric biosensor with human CYP3A4 as a novel drug screening tool," *Biochemical pharmacology,* vol. 65, pp. 1817–1826, 2003.
21. R. Levy, R. Dana, B. Gold, M. Alkan, and F. Schlaeffer, "Influence of calcium channel blockers on polymorphonuclear and monocyte bactericidal and fungicidal activity," *Israel journal of medical sciences,* vol. 27, p. 301, 1991.
22. V. V. Shumyantseva, S. Carrara, V. Bavastrello, D. Jason Riley, T. V. Bulko, K. G. Skryabin, *et al.*, "Direct electron transfer between cytochrome P450scc and gold nanoparticles on screen-printed rhodium–graphite electrodes," *Biosensors and Bioelectronics,* vol. 21, pp. 217–222, 2005.
23. V. Erokhin, S. Carrara, H. Amenitch, S. Bernstorff, and C. Nicolini, "Semiconductor nanoparticles for quantum devices," *Nanotechnology,* vol. 9, p. 158, 1998.
24. L. Soleymani, Z. Fang, E. H. Sargent, and S. O. Kelley, "Programming the detection limits of biosensors through controlled nanostructuring," *Nature Nanotechnology,* vol. 4, pp. 844–848, 2009.

25. A. Guiseppi-Elie, C. Lei, and R. H. Baughman, "Direct electron transfer of glucose oxidase on carbon nanotubes," *Nanotechnology,* vol. 13, p. 559, 2002.
26. S. Carrara, V. V. Shumyantseva, A. I. Archakov, and B. Samorì, "Screen-printed electrodes based on carbon nanotubes and cytochrome P450scc for highly sensitive cholesterol biosensors," *Biosensors and Bioelectronics,* vol. 24, pp. 148–150, 2008.
27. M. Zhou, L. Shang, B. Li, L. Huang, and S. Dong, "Highly ordered mesoporous carbons as electrode material for the construction of electrochemical dehydrogenase-and oxidase-based biosensors," *Biosensors and Bioelectronics,* vol. 24, pp. 442–447, 2008.
28. Y. Shao, J. Wang, H. Wu, J. Liu, I. A. Aksay, and Y. Lin, "Graphene based electrochemical sensors and biosensors: a review," *Electroanalysis,* vol. 22, pp. 1027–1036, 2010.
29. C. Boero, S. Carrara, and G. De Micheli, "Sensitivity enhancement by carbon nanotubes: applications to stem cell cultures monitoring," in *Research in Microelectronics and Electronics, 2009. PRIME 2009. Ph. D.*, 2009, pp. 72–75.
30. C. Boero, S. Carrara, G. Del Vecchio, L. Calzà, and G. De Micheli, "Highly sensitive carbon nanotube-based sensing for lactate and glucose monitoring in cell culture," *NanoBioscience, IEEE Transactions on,* vol. 10, pp. 59–67, 2011.
31. C. Boero, S. Carrara, G. Del Vecchio, L. Calzà, and G. De Micheli, "Targeting of multiple metabolites in neural cells monitored by using protein-based carbon nanotubes," *Sensors and Actuators B: Chemical,* vol. 157, pp. 216–224, 2011.
32. S. Carrara, A. Cavallini, V. Erokhin, and G. De Micheli, "Multi-panel drugs detection in human serum for personalized therapy," *Biosensors and Bioelectronics,* vol. 26, pp. 3914–3919, 2011.
33. A. Cavallini, S. Carrara, G. De Micheli, and V. Erokhin, "P450-mediated electrochemical sensing of drugs in human plasma for personalized therapy," in *Ph. D. Research in Microelectronics and Electronics (PRIME), 2010 Conference on,* 2010, pp. 1–4.
34. S. Carrara, L. Bolomey, C. Boero, A. Cavallini, E. Meurville, G. De Micheli, *et al.*, "Remote System for Monitoring Animal Models With Single-Metabolite Bio-Nano-Sensors," 2013.
35. S. Carrara, A. Cavallini, S. Ghoreishizadeh, J. Olivo, and G. De Micheli, "Developing highly-integrated subcutaneous biochips for remote monitoring of human metabolism," in *Sensors, 2012 IEEE,* 2012, pp. 1–4.
36. G. Wohlfahrt, S. Witt, J. Hendle, D. Schomburg, H. M. Kalisz, and H.-J. Hecht, "1.8 and 1.9 A resolution structures of the Penicillium amagasakiense and Aspergillus niger glucose oxidases as a basis for modelling substrate complexes," *Acta Crystallographica Section D: Biological Crystallography,* vol. 55, pp. 969–977, 1999.
37. C. Baj-Rossi, G. D. Micheli, and S. Carrara, "Electrochemical detection of anti-breast-cancer agents in human serum by cytochrome P450-coated carbon nanotubes," *Sensors,* vol. 12, pp. 6520–6537, 2012.
38. D. M. G. Cavallini Andrea, Carrara Sandro, "Comparison of Three Methods of Biocompatible Multi-Walled Carbon Nanotubes Confinement for the Development of Implantable Amperometric ATP Biosensors," *Sensor Letters,* vol. B 157 pp. 216– 224, 2011.
39. B. J. Gu and J. S. Wiley, "Rapid ATP-induced release of matrix metalloproteinase 9 is mediated by the P2X7 receptor," *Blood,* vol. 107, pp. 4946–4953, 2006.
40. H. Zhu and M. Snyder, "Protein chip technology," *Current opinion in chemical biology,* vol. 7, pp. 55–63, 2003.
41. C. Boero, S. Carrara, and G. De Micheli, "New technologies for nanobiosensing and their applications to real-time monitoring," in *Biomedical Circuits and Systems Conference (BioCAS), 2011 IEEE,* 2011, pp. 357–360.
42. M. Kumar and Y. Ando, "Chemical vapor deposition of carbon nanotubes: a review on growth mechanism and mass production," *Journal of nanoscience and nanotechnology,* vol. 10, pp. 3739–3758, 2010.
43. I. Taurino, S. Carrara, M. Giorcelli, A. Tagliaferro, and G. De Micheli, "Comparing sensitivities of differently oriented multi-walled carbon nanotubes integrated on silicon wafer for electrochemical biosensors," *Sensors and Actuators B: Chemical,* vol. 160, pp. 327–333, 2011.
44. C. Soldano, A. Mahmood, and E. Dujardin, "Production, properties and potential of graphene," *Carbon,* vol. 48, pp. 2127–2150, 2010.

45. A. M. Irene Taurino, Federico Matteini, Lászl6 Forró, Giovanni De Micheli, Sandro Carrara, "Direct growth of nanotubes and graphene nanoflowers on electrochemical platinum electrodes," *Nanoscale,* p. submitted, 2013.
46. D. Johnson, B. Lewis, D. Elliot, J. Miners, and L. Martin, "Electrochemical characterisation of the human cytochrome P450 CYP2C9," *Biochemical pharmacology,* vol. 69, pp. 1533–1541, 2005.
47. R. B. Weiss, R. M. Rifkin, F. M. Stewart, R. L. Theriault, L. A. Williams, A. A. Herman, *et al.*, "High-dose chemotherapy for high-risk primary breast cancer: an on-site review of the Bezwoda study," *The Lancet,* vol. 355, pp. 999–1003, 2000.
48. A. Chang, L. Hui, R. Asbury, L. Boros, G. Garrow, and J. Rubins, "Ifosfamide, carboplatin and etoposide (ICE) in metastatic and refractory breast cancer," *Cancer chemotherapy and pharmacology,* vol. 44, pp. S26–S28, 1999.
49. M. Ayers, W. Symmans, J. Stec, A. Damokosh, E. Clark, K. Hess, *et al.*, "Gene expression profiles predict complete pathologic response to neoadjuvant paclitaxel and fluorouracil, doxorubicin, and cyclophosphamide chemotherapy in breast cancer," *Journal of Clinical Oncology,* vol. 22, pp. 2284–2293, 2004.
50. M. Kaufmann, G. Von Minckwitz, R. Smith, V. Valero, L. Gianni, W. Eiermann, *et al.*, "International expert panel on the use of primary (preoperative) systemic treatment of operable breast cancer: review and recommendations," *Journal of clinical oncology,* vol. 21, pp. 2600–2608, 2003.
51. G. D. M. Camilla Baj-Rossi, Sandro Carrara,, "A Linear Approach to Multi-Panel Sensing in Personalized Therapy for Cancer Treatment," *IEEE Sensor Journal,* p. submitted, 2013.
52. G. De Micheli, S. S. Ghoreishizadeh, C. Boero, F. Valgimigli, and S. Carrara, "An integrated platform for advanced diagnostics," in *Design, Automation & Test in Europe Conference & Exhibition (DATE), 2011,* 2011, pp. 1–6.
53. K. Iniewski, *VLSI circuits for biomedical applications*: Artech House, 2008.
54. H. S. Narula and J. G. Harris, "A time-based VLSI potentiostat for ion current measurements," *Sensors Journal, IEEE,* vol. 6, pp. 239–247, 2006.
55. J. L. Hennessy and D. A. Patterson, *Computer architecture: a quantitative approach*: Morgan Kaufmann, 2011.
56. P. Horowitz, W. Hill, and T. C. Hayes, *The art of electronics* vol. 2: Cambridge university press Cambridge, 1989.
57. A. Cavallini, C. Baj-Rossi, S. Ghoreishizadeh, G. De Micheli, and S. Carrara, "Design, fabrication, and test of a sensor array for perspective biosensing in chronic pathologies," in *Biomedical Circuits and Systems Conference (BioCAS), 2012 IEEE,* 2012, pp. 124–127.
58. C. F. Lee and P. K. Mok, "A monolithic current-mode CMOS DC-DC converter with on-chip current-sensing technique," *Solid-State Circuits, IEEE Journal of,* vol. 39, pp. 3–14, 2004.
59. S. S. Ghoreishizadeh, S. Carrara, and G. De Micheli, Circuit Design for Human Metabolites Biochip, Conference IEEE BioCAS 2011, San Diego, USA, November 10-12, 2011, pp. 460–463
60. P. Schvan, D. Pollex, and T. Bellingrath, "A 22GS/s 6b DAC with integrated digital ramp generator," in *Solid-State Circuits Conference, 2005. Digest of Technical Papers. ISSCC. 2005 IEEE International,* 2005, pp. 122–588.
61. S. S. Ghoreishizadeh, S. Carrara, and G. De Micheli, "Circuit design for human metabolites biochip," in *Biomedical Circuits and Systems Conference (BioCAS), 2011 IEEE,* 2011, pp. 460–463.
62. J. Olivo, S. Carrara, and G. De Micheli, "IronIC patch: A wearable device for the remote powering and connectivity of implantable systems," in *Instrumentation and Measurement Technology Conference (I2MTC), 2012 IEEE International,* 2012, pp. 286–289.
63. S. S. Ghoreishizadeh, I. Taurino, S. Carrara, and G. De Micheli, "A current-mode potentiostat for multi-target detection tested with different lactate biosensors," in *Biomedical Circuits and Systems Conference (BioCAS), 2012 IEEE,* 2012, pp. 128–131.
64. J. Olivo, S. Carrara, and G. De Micheli, "A Study of Multi-Layer Spiral Inductors for Remote Powering of Implantable Sensors," *Biomedical Circuits and Systems, IEEE Transactions on,* vol. in press, 2013.

65. A. S. Poon, S. O'Driscoll, and T. H. Meng, "Optimal frequency for wireless power transmission into dispersive tissue," *Antennas and Propagation, IEEE Transactions on,* vol. 58, pp. 1739–1750, 2010.
66. J. Olivo, S. Carrara, and G. De Micheli, "Optimal frequencies for inductive powering of fully implantable biosensors for chronic and elderly patients," in *Sensors, 2010 IEEE*, 2010, pp. 99–103.
67. B. Datta and W. Burleson, "Circuit-level NBTI macro-models for collaborative reliability monitoring," in *Proceedings of the 20th symposium on Great lakes symposium on VLSI*, 2010, pp. 453–458.
68. C. C. Tan, H. Wang, S. Zhong, and Q. Li, "Body sensor network security: an identity-based cryptography approach," in *Proceedings of the first ACM conference on Wireless network security*, 2008, pp. 148–153.

Chapter 5
In Vivo Bioreactor: New Type of Implantable Medical Devices

Qiang Tan

Tissue Engineering and Regenerative Medicine

Since ancient times, we human beings have dreamed of creating our own tissue and organ substitutes. The oldest version of the dream dates back to the Bible, where it is mentioned that God took a rib from Adam to create Eve.

Here is the latest version: scientists harvest cells from a human being (most often from the bone marrow of a rib, coincidentally) and expand them in vitro before seeding them onto a biodegradable scaffold that is shaped according to the contours of the tissue to be replaced. The cell-scaffold construct is then cultured in a so-called bioreactor, a device that mimics the in vivo regenerative niche. As is often seen in science fiction movies, the living organ substitute is always immersed in some magic liquid with various growth factors to induce tissue formation before being implanted in a human body.

This technique, referred to as tissue engineering by Langer and Vacanti in the 1990s, epitomizes the unprecedented achievements from stem cell research, cell therapy, biomaterial science, and genetic engineering. It represents the state of the art of regenerative medicine [1]. To the public, tissue engineering remained a crazy dream of some eccentric scientists until 1997, when Dr. Yilin Cao showed a human ear regenerated on the back of a nude mouse [2]. The ear immediately attracted the attention of everyone who simply believed it would be a piece of cake to remove the ear from the mouse for human clinical application. More than a dozen years and billions of investment dollars later, the ear remains on the back of the nude mouse. What went wrong?

With the enthusiasm gone, it is time to contemplate the disadvantages and technical obstacles inherent in the conventional tissue-engineering process:

Q. Tan (✉)
The Department of Thoracic Surgery, Shanghai Chest Hospital, Shanghai, China
e-mail: tqiang@hotmail.com

W. Burleson and S. Carrara (eds.), *Security and Privacy for Implantable Medical Devices*,
DOI 10.1007/978-1-4614-1674-6_5,

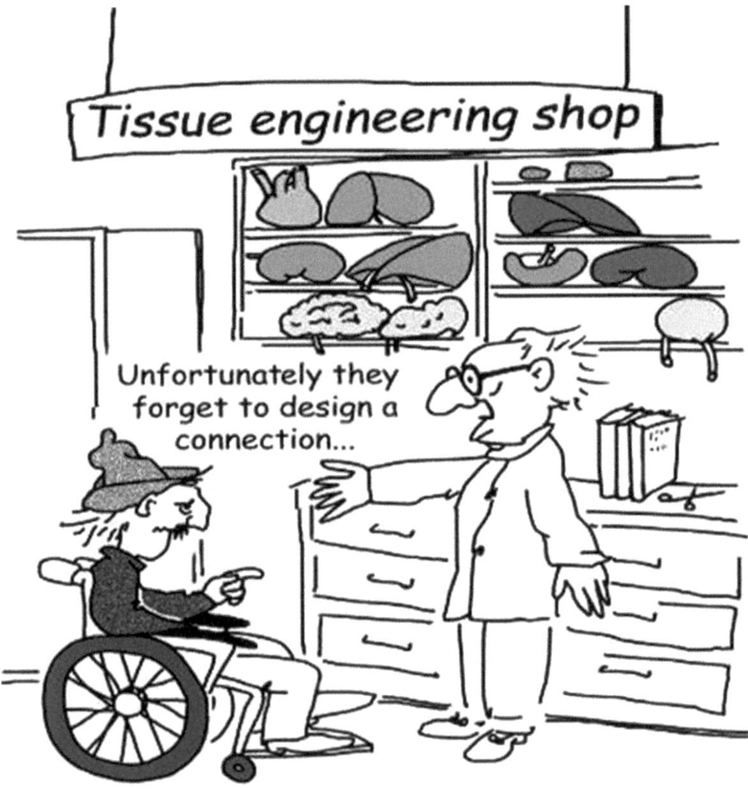

Fig. 5.1 Revascularization remains the key obstacle to tissue engineering technique clinic application

(i) Problems with the traditional tissue-engineering procedure: traditional tissue-engineering techniques were composed of two absolutely separate stages, in vitro three-dimensional (3D) culture of the tissue-engineered (TE) substitute and in vivo regeneration of the implanted substitute. This technique relied on the hope that the vascular system could also be reconstructed in vitro inside the TE substitute, which could also be easily connected to the recipient's circulation, as is the case in organ transplantation (Fig. 5.1). Unfortunately, it proved to be extremely difficult, if not impossible, to rebuild the capillary vessels in the TE organ in vitro [3, 4]. Previous studies proved that implanted substitutes depended for nutrition on tissue fluid infiltration and vessel ingrowth from the surrounding tissue. Unfortunately, this revascularization process normally took several weeks. The central part of the TE substitute would suffer from ischemia right after implantation, leading to the death of the majority of preseeded cells and poison the regenerative niche [5, 6]. This fact brought into questioning the necessity of cell preseeding and giving birth to the in situ tissue engineering theory, which neglected cells and implanted only the shaped biodegradable scaffold together with growth factor(s) to induce in situ stem cell growth and differentiation [7, 8]. This modification was not very successful and demonstrated the critical function of cells in the regenerative process. Considering the fact that we age because of a decreased capacity for stem cell proliferation, it should not be surprising that we need cells for truly functional reconstruction. Delayed revascularization kills most cells within implanted constructs and prevents the clinical application of large TE prostheses. So far, successful clinical application of TE products has only been accomplished in cartilage tissue (which is avascular) and skin (which is placed on a well-vascularized wound surface) [9, 10].

(ii) Problems with bioreactor: for traditional tissue engineering, a bioreactor mimicking the in vivo regenerative niche was critical for in vitro 3D tissue and organ reconstruction [11, 12]. Ironically, our knowledge of specific tissue and organ regeneration was too limited to prevent cell dedifferentiation and to allow various kinds of cells maintaining the 3D organization associated with normal organ structure [13, 14]. This was the rarely known reason why scientists had to culture the human-ear-shaped cartilage tissue first on the back of a nude mouse, which functioned as a living in vivo bioreactor, before moving it to the human body. However, even if the bioreactor precisely presented the in vivo regenerative niche, the well-nourished cells located at the surface of the scaffold would proliferate quickly and form a dense tissue layer preventing the infiltration of nutrients into the central part of the TE substitute, leading to a hollow structure with only scaffold and dead cells in the central part [15]. This would surely compromise the mechanical strength and biocompatibility of the TE substitute. Poor knowledge of regenerative niches and the limitation of nutrient infiltration into the substitute prevented us from making the Hollywood style dreams of culture-organ-in-bottles come true.

(iii) Problems with in vivo regeneration: After implantation, the TE substitute went through regenerative and revascularization processes to become compatible to the recipient. The final regenerated tissue and organ proved to be a hybrid of preseeded cells and in situ regenerative cells [16]. When scientist tried to repeat their successful nude-mouse-human-ear project on a rabbit or sheep model, the immune system of the recipients, unlike that of the nude mouse, were strongly activated by the biodegradable scaffold and dead cells in the "hollow-structured" TE substitute. Ultimately, the whole substitute was absorbed, leaving only granulation tissue. No matter how well organized cells were inside the prosthesis, after implantation they would be reorganized during the revascularization process to integrate into the recipient [17]. Similar to fixing a car with the accessories from an abandoned old car which required to be disassembled first, the interaction between recipient and TE prosthesis is a process of destruction and reorganization based on a 3D scaffold to provide the structure and enough living cells to guarantee functional reconstruction. Moreover, biocompatibility is obviously a key issue for successful regeneration.

(iv) Problems with growth factors: Various growth factors constitute the regenerative niche and are often lacking in damaged tissue [18, 19]. In almost all bioreactor designs, we emphasized the importance of standard medium without serum during the entire in vitro 3D substitute culture process and neglected the spatial and temporal model of various grow factor combinations. Just imagine the consequences if you decided to feed your children with the best milk possible for his/her whole life. Meanwhile it is difficult to control growth factor concentration at the site of regeneration in vivo. Gene transfection and growth factor integration into biomaterials are technically demanding and not efficient [20, 21]. How to keep the effective growth factor concentration inside TE prosthesis is therefore another technical obstacle to successful clinical application of tissue engineering.

To summarize, we seem to know all the requirements for tissue and organ regeneration: the cells, the biodegradable scaffold, and the growth factors. However, we have failed to organize the three essential elements well enough to perfectly interact with the recipient by matching and, to some extent, promoting the natural regenerative process.

The In Vivo Bioreactor

Perhaps it is time to compromise on the dream of creating tissue and organ substitutes exclusively in vitro. Since implanted TE substitutes will undergo a hybrid process with surrounding tissue and our understanding of the regenerative niche in vivo is not crystal clear, it might make sense to take advantage of the recipients' own regenerative power for the reconstruction of their own tissue and organ substitutes. To that end, we propose a so-called in vivo bioreactor design, which may be described as implanted TE substitutes perfused with an intrascaffold flow of medium created by an extracorporeal portable pump system for in situ tissue and organ regeneration [22]. This design combines the traditionally separated in vitro 3D cell-scaffold culture system and the in vivo regenerative processes associated with TE substitutes, while treating the recipients as bioreactors for their TE prostheses. Three main functions have been demonstrated during our pilot experiments on TE trachea with this in vivo bioreactor design [23].

The trachea has become one of the hot topics in tissue-engineering research mainly due to a misunderstanding that treated the trachea as no more than a tubular cartilage conduit [22, 24]. Since cartilage tissue is avascular, researchers wrongly believed that they could ignore the revascularization obstacle of tissue engineering. Unfortunately, the whole history of trachea replacement has emphasized the importance of an intact epithelial layer covering the inner tracheal lumen, which prevents both bacterial invasion and granulation tissue overgrowth [25]. Since the epithelial layer depends on a well-vascularized submucosal layer for nutrition, we must still face the revascularization problem when reconstructing the trachea using a tissue-engineering technique. Professor Belsey, a pioneer in trachea surgery, stated that "the intrathoracic portion of the trachea is the last unpaired organ in the body to fall to the surgeon, and the successful solution of the problem of its reconstruction may mark the end of the 'expansionist' epoch in the development of surgery" [26]. This pertinent statement makes the trachea a typical sample for novel tissue-engineering research.

To prove the principle, we first established an in vitro model of the in vivo bioreactor to test its efficiency in supporting cell survival and function as a cell seeding and growth factor delivery system [23].

Description of the "In Vivo Bioreactor" Test Model

To assemble a simple test model of the in vivo bioreactor, we chose a biodegradable tubular polyesterurethanes (DegraPol) scaffold (provided by Dr. P. Neuenschwander, Institute of Polymer Research ETHZ, Zurich, Switzerland), 2 cm in length and 2 mm in inner diameter [27]. A catheter (6 F angiographic catheter, 1 mm inner diameter, Cordis, Spreitenbach, Switzerland) was inserted into the lumen of the DegraPol tube. Half of the catheter wall located inside the DegraPol lumen was cut to allow the medium to leak out and filtrate into the scaffold. Each end of the catheter was connected to a peristaltic pump (IPC high-precision, multichannel dispenser, ISMATEC, Zurich, Switzerland). One pump continuously supplied the perfusate into the scaffold, while the other drained the waste (Fig. 5.2a, b). Both ran at a speed of 5 mL/h.

Epithelial Cell Survival Test

Survival Test

Since an intact epithelial layer is a prerequisite for a successful trachea substitute and the epithelium is more sensitive to ischemia than chondrocytes, we chose to use epithelium for a cell survival test. A porcine split-thickness (200 μm) skin graft was wrapped around the tubular DegraPol scaffold of the in vivo bioreactor test model and perfused with medium at 10 mL/h for 1 week. In the control group, the tubular DegraPol covered with a skin graft was immersed in the medium with the epithelial layer exposed to the air. After 1 week, the histology results showed a living epithelial layer with an intact basement membrane in the in vivo bioreactor group, while the epithelial layer and dermis were completely separated in the control group (Fig. 5.3).

Based on this result, we hypothesized that in the in vivo bioreactor group, the medium flow increased the infiltration pressure and made the nutrients penetrate deeper enough into the skin graft to support the survival of the basal stem cells on the basement membrane [28, 29]. Furthermore, the basal stem cells proliferated to form a multilayered epithelium and maintain the intact basement membrane, thereby preventing dermis granulation tissue overgrowth. To demonstrate this hypothesis, we compared the partial tissue oxygen tension (tPO_2) by polarographic microprobes and measured the metabolic activity (via glucose and lactate levels) by microdialysis at different thicknesses inside the TE skin with and without perfusion [30]. Perfluorocarbon-based artificial oxygen carriers were chosen to mimic the hemoglobin in blood [31].

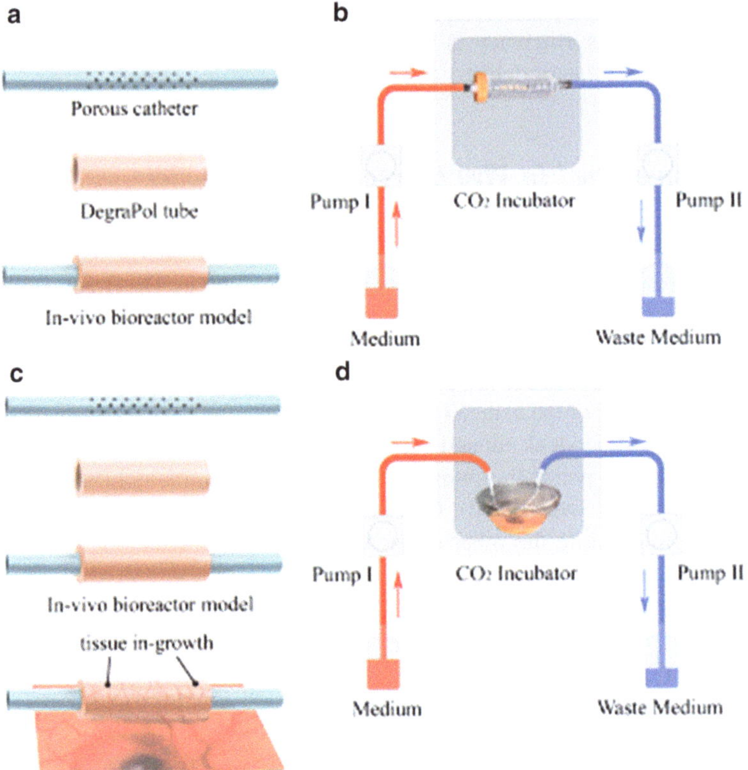

Fig. 5.2 In vivo bioreactor test model and angiogenesis test on chicken chorioallantoic membrane (CAM). (**a**) Porous catheter inserted into tubular DegraPol tube. (**b**) The porous catheter was connected to two peristaltic pumps, which created a flow of medium passing through the cather and penetrating into the DegraPol scaffold preserved in a centrifuge tube inside a CO_2 incubator. Unlike traditional bioreactor designs, which immerse the biodegradable scaffold (DegraPol scaffold in this model) inside media, the "in vivo bioreactor" testing model creates a flow of medium inside the scaffold. (**c**) The "in vivo bioreactor" testing model was placed on the surface of CAM, presenting the normal tissue surrounding the tissue-engineered prosthesis. (**d**) "In vivo bioreactor" testing model placed on CAM was used as a testing model for the revascularization process of tissue-engineered prosthesis

Tissue Oxygen Tension and Metabolism Test

The human tracheal epithelial cell line, 16HBE14o, was cultured and seeded onto xenogenic (porcine) acellular dermal matrices (ADMs) at a concentration of $1 \times 10*7$/mL [32]. Two hours after cell seeding, the cell-scaffold constructs were cultured at the air–liquid interface in six-well Transwell permeable supports for 1 week. During the tPO_2 measurement, the TE epithelium was folded to pinch the polarographic microprobes within the epithelium before putting it on the surface of a porous rectangular poly(ethylene oxide terephthalate)-poly(butylene terephthalate) (PEOT/PBT) scaffold [33].

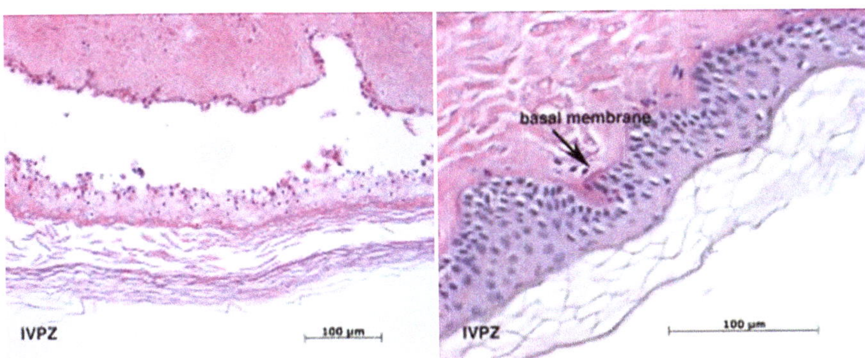

Fig. 5.3 The histology results showed that the epithelial layer and dermis was completely separated in the control group (*on the left,*) while the living epithelial layer with an intact basement membrane was detected in the in vivo bioreactor group (*on the right*)

A continuous flow of medium was created inside the PEOT/PBT scaffold through two inserted needles each of whose ends were connected to a peristaltic pump via Tygon long flex life (LFL) tubes. The inlet pump delivered medium continuously into the scaffold, while the outlet pump sucked the waste out. To prevent oxygen exchange between the intrascaffold medium and air during the tPO_2 measurement, the TE trachea patch under perfusion was wrapped within rat skin (Fig. 5.4). Normal Dulbecco's modified Eagle's medium (DMEM) and Oxygent^{TM} DMEM reoxygenated with air or pure oxygen were sequentially used as perfusate.

Epithelial tPO_2 was assessed with Clark-type microprobes consisting of polarographic electrodes and an oxygen-sensitive microcell (Revoxode CC1, Integra Kiel, UK). The TE epithelial tissue was folded, and one polarographic microprobe was pinched within the fold to guarantee that the results would reflect the oxygen pressure level inside the epithelial tissue. Another polarographic microprobe was inserted between the TE epithelium and the rat skin that wrapped around the whole TE trachea patch. These two polarographic microprobes measured the oxygen distribution within the epithelial tissue at different thicknesses. The proximal one pinched within the folded TE epithelial tissue was around 200 μm (the thickness of ADM) above the medium, while the distal one was at double the thickness, or 400 μm. During the measurement, six TE trachea patch samples were randomly assigned to two groups, which were perfused with either DMEM or Oxygent^{TM} DMEM as follows: (i) perfusion for 30 min, (ii) stop perfusion for 30 min, (iii) restart perfusion for 30 min. The perfusates were then reoxygenated with 100% oxygen for 10 min, and the perfusion procedure was repeated. All the measurements were performed in an incubator at 37°C with 5% CO_2.

The epithelium tPO_2 measurement results are summarized in Fig. 5.5, with two curves in each picture representing the changes in tPO_2 under perfusion of DMEM and Oxygent^{TM} DMEM, respectively. Each curve can be separated into three parts: Phase I reflects the TE trachea epithelium tPO_2 level under stable continuous

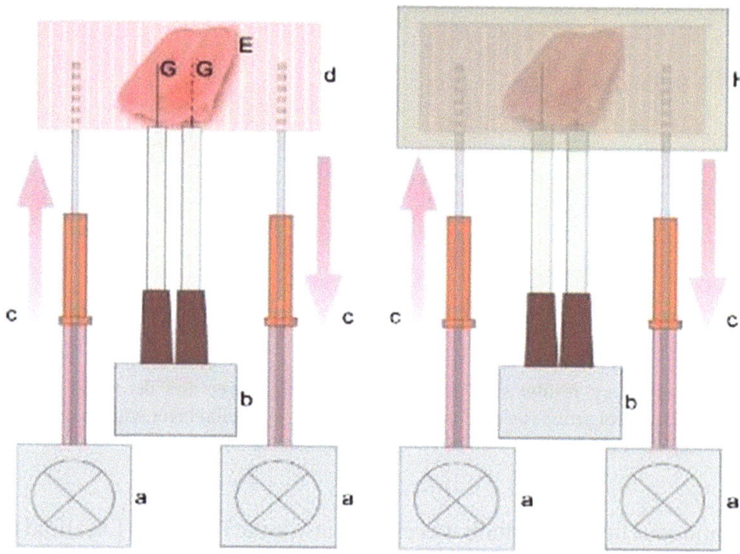

Fig. 5.4 Sketch for the epithelial tissue partial oxygen tension (tPO_2) measurement setting. (**a**) Peristaltic pump. (**b**) Polarographic microprobes. (**c**) Perfusion of medium inside the re-epithelialized tissue-engineered trachea patch. (**d**) Porous rectangular poly(ethylene oxide terephthalate)-poly(butylene terephthalate) (PEOT/PBT) scaffold. E:Tissue-engineered epithelium. G:Probes for tPO_2 measurement, one pinched within the tissue epithelium, with the other on the surface. H:rat skin used to cover the re-epithelialized tissue-engineered trachea patch, preventing air exchange with air

medium perfusion, Phase II represents the decrease in tPO_2 after the perfusion was stopped; and Phase III depicts the increase in tPO_2 after the medium perfusion was restarted.

Epithelial metabolism was measured by microdialysis probes (CMA/20, CMA Microdialysis, Kista, Sweden) with a molecular weight cutoff of 20,000 Da and membrane length of 5 mm [34]. Six pieces of TE trachea epithelium were randomly assigned to DMEM and Oxygent™ DMEM perfusion groups. The TE trachea epithelium was folded to pinch the microdialysis probe and put on top of the PEOT/PBT scaffold perfused with DMEM or Oxygent™ DMEM as described earlier. In contrast, the whole setting was not enveloped in rat skin due to the fact that tracheal epithelium is physiologically exposed to the air. The probes were equilibrated for 1 h followed by continuous measurements of epithelial glucose, lactate, and pyruvate concentrations for 8 h. The TE trachea epithelium metabolite concentrations under different medium perfusions for 8 h are summarized in Fig. 5.6.

All these results indicated that in the in vivo bioreactor design, where oxygen was transported into the TE prosthesis by both diffusion and convection, we were able to support the survival of 200-μm-thick epithelial tissue. In contrast, in static culture, where the oxygen was transported by diffusion only, tissue no more than 100 μm could form.

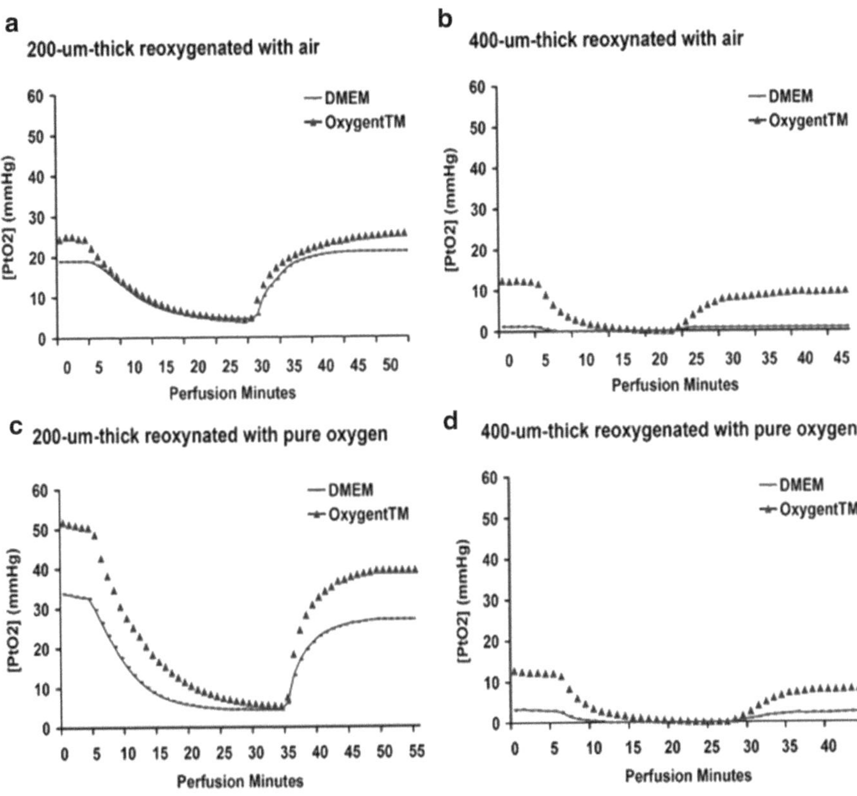

Fig. 5.5 Under continuous perfusion with DMEM reoxygenated by air, the tPO_2 level stabilized around 18.8 ± 0.1 mmHg at the proximal part (200 μm thickness) and 1.1 ± 0.1 mmHg at the distal part (400 μm thickness) of TE trachea epithelium. The corresponding data under Oxygent™ DMEM perfusion were 23.7 ± 0.7 mmHg and 11.8 ± 0.5 mmHg, respectively, and both showed significant difference in comparison with DMEM perfusion data ($\rho < 0.01$). After we stopped the pump, the tPO_2 levels declined at similar rates in both groups to 4.67 ± 0.07 mmHg at the proximal part; at the distal part, the tPO_2 dropped precipitously within 3 min to 0 mmHg in the DMEM perfusion group, while this process lasted for nearly 20 min in the Oxygent™ perfusion group. The bottom number in Phase II actually represents the tPO_2 level in static culture. When we restarted the perfusion, the tPO_2 level resumed at a rate around 15.50 mmHg/min proximally and 0.08 mmHg/min distally in the DMEM group. In the Oxygent™ DMEM perfusion group, the resume rate was similar at the proximal part (around 17.50 mmHg/min), while almost ten times faster at the distal part (0.81 mmHg/min) than the resume rate of DMEM perfusion group. By comparing the area under Phase II, we concluded that tissue-engineered epithelial tissue under the Oxygent™ DMEM perfusion gained 10.34% more at the proximal part and 3427.44% more at the distal part than that under DMEM perfusion. Under continuous perfusion with DMEM reoxygenated with pure oxygen, the TE epithelium tPO_2 level reached 33.2 ± 0.2 mmHg proximally and 3.1 ± 0.01 mmHg distally; the level dropped to 5.5 ± 0.1 mmHg within 15 min and 0 mmHg within 5 min, respectively, after we stopped the perfusion pump. The tPO_2 level resumed at 21.40 mmHg/min proximally and 0.21 mmHg/min distally when we restarted the perfusion. With respect to the Oxygent™ DMEM group, the tPO2 level was 51.0 ± 0.3 mmHg proximally and 12.4 ± 0.1 mmHg distally under continuous perfusion; it dropped to 5.5 ± 0.1 mmHg in 25 min

The continuous flow of medium inside the cell-scaffold construct could support the survival of cells and their ability to form 200-μm-thick 3D microtissue on the surface of the scaffold, which is critical to maintaining their normal function. This microtissue will be reorganized to contribute to regeneration, which features the in-growth of vessels from the surrounding tissue. This experiment also demonstrated the feasibility of using simple, readily applicable, and nondestructive implanted biosensors to monitor the regenerative process of TE substitutes in situ, allowing for early warning of inappropriate changes in cell metabolic activity [35–37]. The in vivo bioreactor design also provide us with an approach to making timely adjustment to cells survive and thrive, as well as to maintaining the normal regenerative niche.

Chondrocyte Seeding Test

According to traditional tissue-engineering protocol, the cell-scaffold construct is cultured in vitro for several months to form a mature tissue for implantation. Unfortunately, this kind of delay is not acceptable for most emergency trauma operations. Furthermore, other drawbacks make this protocol unreasonable in practice.

The first drawback relates to the fact that we are unable to create a vascular system inside a TE prosthesis that can be directly connected to the recepient's circulatory system, as is the case in organ transplantation, to nourish the seeded cells. After implantation, the TE prosthesis depends on the in-growth of a capillary network from surrounding host tissues to secure nutrient supply. Unfortunately, the revascularization process normally takes months. As a direct result, 99% of preseeded cells inside a TE prothesis die of ischemia and toxicity within the regenerative niche. The delayed revascularization frustrates the effort used for in vitro cell seeding and culture [38].

Secondly, in the traditional tissue-engineering protocol the optimal implant time needs to be properly defined. For example, for a TE trachea, a partially developed cell-scaffold construct facilitates the revascularization process but provides inadequate mechanical strength. On the other hand, a long-term cultured, mature TE trachea is strong enough to prevent collapse but hinders blood vessel in-growth after implantation [39].

Fig. 5.5 (Continued) and 0 mmHg in 20 min, respectively; it resumed at a rate around 29.5 mmHg/min proximally and 0.76 mmHg/min distally within 15 min. There were significant differences regarding the tPO_2 level and change rates in all three phases between DMEM and Oxygent^{TM} DMEM perfusion groups, both proximally and distally of the TE epithelium. By measuring the area under Phase II, we found the TE trachea epithelium oxygen content under Oxygent^{TM} DMEM perfusion to be 73.79% more in the proximal part and 607.22% more in the distal part than that under DMEM perfusion

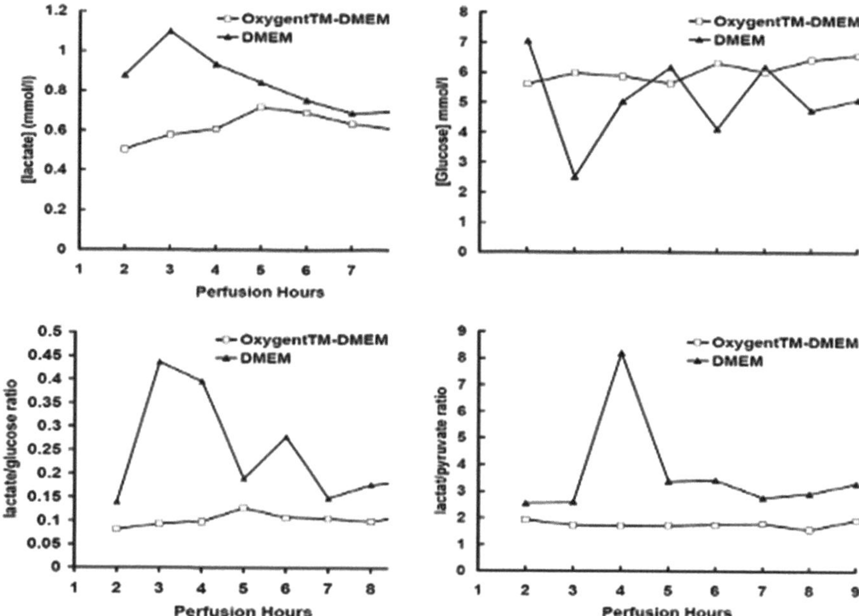

Fig. 5.6 The even curve of the Oxygent^{TM} group indicated a homeostasis niche of TE epithelium under Oxygent^{TM} perfusion. Accordingly, statistical analysis showed a significant increase in the DMEM perfusion group of lactate concentration (0.632 ± 0.005 vs. 0.825 ± 0.021 mmol/L, $\rho < 0.01$), lactate/pyruvate ratio (1.776 ± 0.014 vs. 3.649 ± 3.484, $\rho < 0.05$), and lactate/glucose ratio (0.103 ± 0.000 vs. 0.244 ± 0.013, $\rho < 0.01$). The glucose concentration remained similar (6.062 ± 0.129 vs. 5.124 ± 1.988, $\rho > 0.05$) between both groups, although the data variance of the Oxygent^{TM} perfusion group was much smaller (0.129 vs. 1.989)

Thirdly, a large amount of cells are required in the traditional tissue-engineering protocol. To obtain enough cells, primary cells are often proliferated for several passages before seeding onto the scaffold. Previous studies proved that cells would dedifferentiate after around five passages in vitro in an unnatural niche, leading to a shortage of cells and possible repeated biopsy to obtain more primary cells. Similarly, after being seeded onto a scaffold, most cells also dedifferentiated after long-term culture and failed to secrete a normal extracellular matrix to maintain tissue structure and function [40–42]. All these facts compromise the clinical application of tissue engineering. In contrast, the in vivo biorector design integrates the in vitro reconstruction and in vivo regeneration stages. In an emergency case, the scaffold could be implanted without preseeded cells and at the same time the tissue could be harvested for later isolation and expansion of appropriate autologous cells in the laboratory. The cultured cells could then be harvested and added to the perfusate to be seeded into the implanted scaffolds through daily transfusions. In our opinion, this should be a physiological and economical way to construct TE prostheses while avoiding overproliferation and overseeding of cells. Also, the in

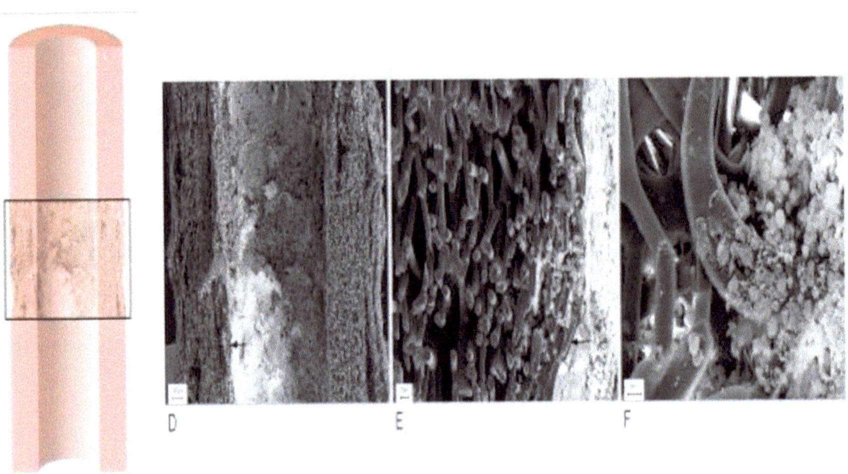

Fig. 5.7 Scanning electron microscope (SEM) images showed that chondrocytes attached and migrated into the DegraPol scaffold in the in vivo biorector seeding test model

vivo bioreactor design would prevent excessive damage resulting from harvesting primary cells from recipients, who would function as bioreactors to the cell-scaffold construct.

To prove the principle using the previous model, we tested the possibility of combining cell seeding and 3D culture systems with the in vivo bioreactor [43]. The aim of this study was to test the possibility of seeding chondrocytes onto DegraPol scaffolds by means of continuous intrascaffold flow of medium and compare the perfusion culture with traditional static culture. In tissue-engineering research, many studies have focused on the establishment of efficient cell-seeding approaches and the optimization of cell culture systems in order to obtain an even distribution of vital cells inside scaffolds [44–46]. During pilot studies, we mixed one flask of chondrocytes with 250 mL medium and tried to seed the cells onto the scaffold through continuous perfusion. Unfortunately, we hardly found any cells attached to the scaffold due to low medium cell concentration and insufficient time for cells to migrate and attach to the scaffold. As a result, we chose to use a semidynamic seeding procedure involving the injection of 1 mL of highly concentrated cell perfusate through the perfusion catheter, followed by a 2 h pause to allow for cell adhesion before restarting perfusion. With this approach, a better 3D cell growth was observed compared with traditional cell seeding of static cultures (Fig. 5.7). Similar to several other studies, the MTT (3-(4,5-Dimethylthiazol-2-yl)-2,5-diphenyltetrazolium bromide); GAG (glycosaminoglycan) results demonstrated that medium perfusion could increase cell content and matrix synthesis in 3D cell culture systems [47, 48].

In contrast to the static culture group, where the chondrocytes only formed a monolayer on the surface of the DegraPol scaffold, our experiment showed

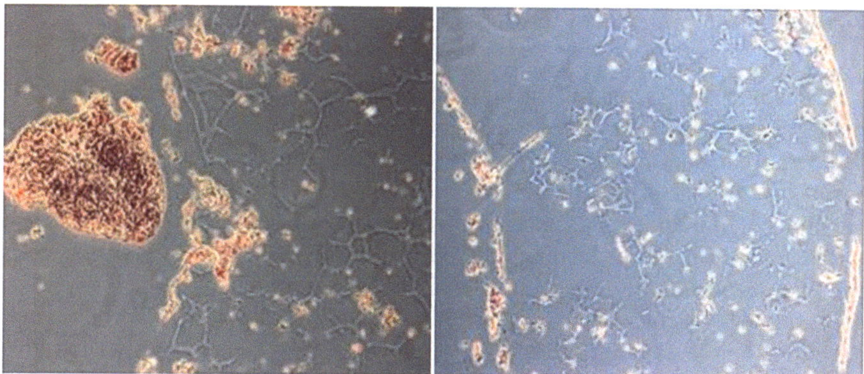

Fig. 5.8 Histology results showed that chondrocytes formed 3D microtissue inside the DegraPol lumen, while chondrocytes only form a monolayer on the DegraPol surface in the static culture group

3D chondrocyte growth forming microtissue in the perfusion culture group. This phenomenon can be well explained by our previous cell survival test findings, which showed that the flowing medium supported much thicker tissue formation than static culture through the combination of diffusion and convention of nutrients and oxygen in the medium (Fig. 5.8).

In addition, our results demonstrated that the in vivo bioreactor design made it possible to avoid using a high concentration of cells for seeding, facilitating the application of TE prostheses in emergency cases. The in vivo bioreactor design provides an opportunity to technically circumvent cell dedifferentiation by extending the seeding of cells throughout the entire regenerative process. Taking the construction of TE trachea as an example, the autologous chondrocytes within limited generations can be seeded into the implanted tissue graft during the entire regeneration period through daily cell transfusion. These cells will contribute to the repair and remodeling of the impaired tissue according to the signaling of the local regenerative niche.

An analogy might help us further understand the benefits of the in vivo bioreactor: we receive a mission to rebuild a unique architecture in a foreign country. Unfortunately, our knowledge of the inner structure and how the architecture was connected to the city to perform normal functions is limited. We only know the building component. Thus, the rational plan would be to provide enough components (cells, growth factors) and maintain their normal function (perfusion to make the cells living). Instead of wasteful building based on our imagination, we should allow the local architect to make good use of all the raw materials and organize them into the appropriate architecture. Following a similar principle, the design of the in vivo bioreactor takes advantage of recipients' own regenerative power, using recipients as bioreactors for the construction of their own TE organs.

Growth Factor Delivery Test

Tissue engineering consists of three core elements: cells, custom-made 3D biodegradable scaffolds, and various growth factors. Being the essence of the regenerative niche, the proper growth factor concentration and the synergy of various growth factors play key roles in tissue reconstruction [49, 50]. Following the protocol of traditional tissue engineering, it proved difficult to keep an efficient concentration of growth factor inside TE prostheses. For example, angiogenesis proved to be a complex process involving various growth factors, which should be applied either together or in sequence [51]. In the case of the in vivo bioreactor, the expression level of different kinds of growth factors can be readily controlled through the adjustment of dose concentration in the perfusate. A detailed spatial and temporal application scheme is also feasible, which has proven to be extremely difficult in other delivery methods, such as gene transfer and growth factor–scaffold binding. To prove this principle, we established an angiogenesis test model. The *ex ovo* chorioallantoic membrane (CAM) model was chosen to test the impact of the in vivo bioreactor system on angiogenesis. On incubation day 8, 16 CAMs were treated as follows. Part of the surface of the CAM membrane was wounded by a tiny drop of alcohol, where a DegraPol tube (1 cm long, 2 mm inner diameter) was then placed. All CAMs were then divided equally and randomly into four groups:

(I) Static control group: 1 cm DegraPol tube only, without medium perfusion.
(II) Vascular endothelial growth factor (VEGF) precoat group: DegraPol tube immersed in a highly concentrated VEGF medium (4,000 ng/mL) without medium perfusion.
(III) In vivo bioreactor group: the porous catheter was connected to perfusion pumps and medium continuously administered through the DegraPol tube.
(V) VEGF perfusion group: same structure as group III, except 40 ng/mL VEGF was added to the perfusion medium

All samples were collected for histological exam after 5 days. One hour before harvest, Bisbenzimide H 33342 (100 μL, 1 μg/mL) was injected into the CAM circulatory system to prove functional vessel formation inside the scaffold [23].

Although the in vivo CAM model has a time limitation in representing the whole process of angiogenesis, we were able to detect erythrocytes migrating all over the scaffold in the samples from group IV (Fig. 5.9). This migration was due to the increased vascular permeability effected by VEGF and neo-vessel formation that occurred much earlier inside the scaffold compared with the control groups. Bisbenzimide H 33342 injection into normal CAM capillary far from the scaffold demonstrated that these vessels within the implant were connected to the embryo's circulation (Fig. 5.10). Through this study, we proved that the in vivo bioreactor could be used as an efficient growth factor delivery system.

To summarize, through an in vitro testing model we proved the three advantages of in vivo bioreactor design. First, it supports the survival of seed cells before integration into the recipient's own regeneration process. Second, it facilitates

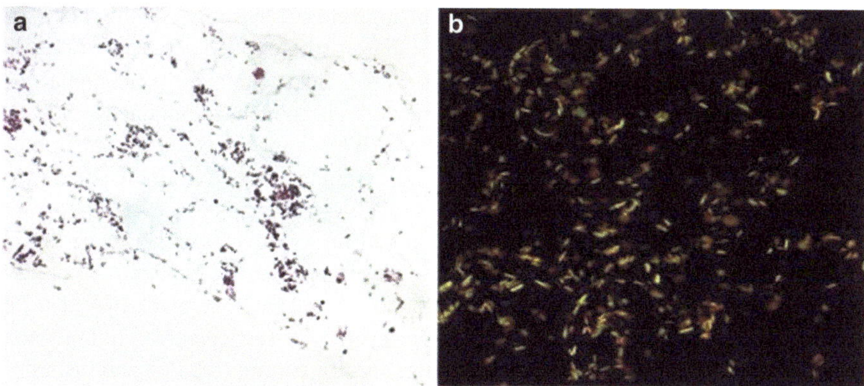

Fig. 5.9 (**a**) Erythrocytes migrated onto the upper part of DegraPol scaffold, which did not come in contact with the CAM tissue. (**b**) The nuclei of erythrocytes were marked brown by H33342 injected into the CAM capillary away from the DegraPol site. This fact proved these erythrocytes migrated from the vessel connected to circulatory system of the embryo

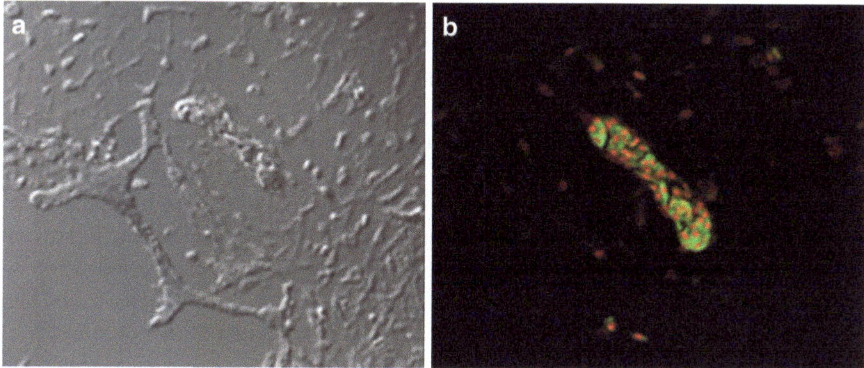

Fig. 5.10 (**a**) CAM tissue with capillary vessels grew into the DegraPol scaffold. (**b**) H33342 marked endothelial nuclei proved the vesselwais connected to the embryo's circulation

a continuous seeding process, avoiding an in vitro high-concentration seeding process. Lastly, it functions as an efficient controllable growth factor delivery system to maintain the local regenerative niche.

Pilot Animal Experiment

In 2008, Dr. Parolo Macchiarini of Barcelona, Spain, published in *The Lancet* the first clinical application of a TE airway [52, 53]. Using an allogenic acellular trachea scaffold seeded with autologous bronchial epithelial cells and chondrocytes induced from bone marrow stromal cells, the Spainish group successfully constructed a TE airway in an InBreath bioreactor. They used the substitute to replace 5 cm of the left main bronchus of a 30-year-old woman suffering from an end-stage bronchomalacia caused by tuberculosis. The result is inspiring. The patient maintained a normal appearance and improved her quality of life with a mechanically reconstructed functional airway. Meanwhile, the authors also frankly announced in the paper that, "although the graft was completely covered with viable mucosa at 1 month, we cannot say whether these cells originated from those seeded or whether they grew in from an adjacent healthy airway," which could be considered a euphemism for "we cannot say whether this was an allogenic acellular trachea transplantation or a TE process, since we were not able to prove the survival of seeded cells." In that case, the TE trachea remains an unsolved problem requiring more research and insight.

Based on the aforementioned in vitro experiment results, we moved forward to a pilot animal experiment using the in vivo bioreactor for a patch repair of a tracheal defect in sheep.

After anesthesia, endotracheal intubation, and ventilation, a 2-cm-long and 1-cm-wide defect was made in the anterior cartilage wall of sheep trachea. Mimicking the normal tracheal structure, the TE tracheal patch was made of three layers: an inner layer consisting of an acellular porcine dermal matrix (submucosal layer); a middle layer consisting of chondrocytes seeded onto a poly(ethylene glycol)–terephthalate-poly(butyleneterephthalate) (PEGT/PBT) scaffold (for the reconstruction of cartilage tissue); and an outer layer consisting of one more acellular porcine dermal matrix (adventitia) to complete a closed system for medium perfusion to follow. The arch-shaped patch was sutured to cover the tracheal defect with around 1 cm overlap over the side walls to strengthen the patch–trachea connection and to prevent collapse during breathing. Two totally implantable venous access devices (Port-a-Caths) were implanted subcutaneously on the back of the neck of the sheep. The catheters of the Port-a-Caths were inserted between the middle and outer layers of the TE tracheal patch.

After the sheep awoke from the operation, each embedded Port-a-Cath was connected to an extracorporeal pump through a Gripper to complete the in vivo bioreactor design (Fig. 5.11). A custom-designed jacket with two separate pockets on the back were put on the sheep. The two pumps were set firmly inside each pocket to allow the sheep to move at liberty without affecting its ability to drink and eat. We chose CADD pumps for our system because they are widely used in the clinic for patients receiving total parenteral nutrition (TPN). One pump administered medium at 10 mL/h into the TE trachea, while the other one simultaneously sucked out the waste at the same speed. Cartilage tissue was harvested during the operation, from which chondrocytes were isolated and subsequently cultured in vitro for three generations. Two weeks after the operation, when the perfusion system remained stable, around 10^7 chondrocytes were harvested, resuspended in 1 cm saline, and injected into the TE tracheal patch through the catheter each day for 1 week. In the control group, the sheep wore the same pump system, while no medium was perfused through the TE tracheal patch (Fig. 5.12).

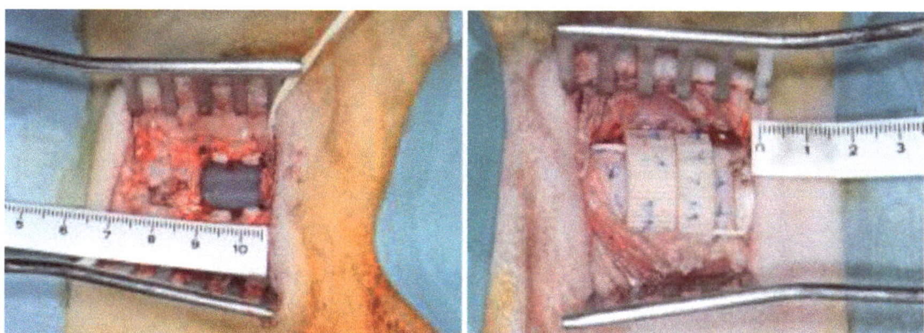

Fig. 5.11 A 2×1 cm defect on the anterior wall of the sheep trachea (*on the left*). This was covered with an acellular porcine dermal matrix and arch-shaped poly(ethylene glycol)–terephthalate-poly(butylene terephthalate) (PEGT/PBT) scaffold, into which Port-a-Cath catheters were inserted

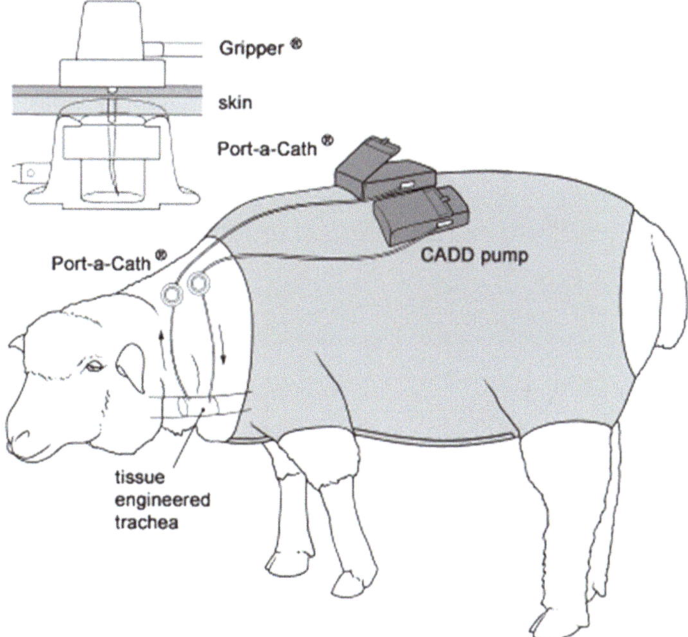

Fig. 5.12 Sketch of the pumping system used in the in vivo bioreactor system for the sheep

In the perfusion group, perfusion only lasted for 1 month before the catheter became blocked. The sheep was sacrificed 3 months after the operation. Gross examination showed the patency of the tracheal lumen was normal, without signs of stenosis caused by granulation tissue overgrowth. Nearly 70% of the PEGT/PBT scaffold did not degrade. In the remaining 30%, we found cartilage tissue formation, which was confirmed by collagen II immunohistochemistry and Safranin O staining.

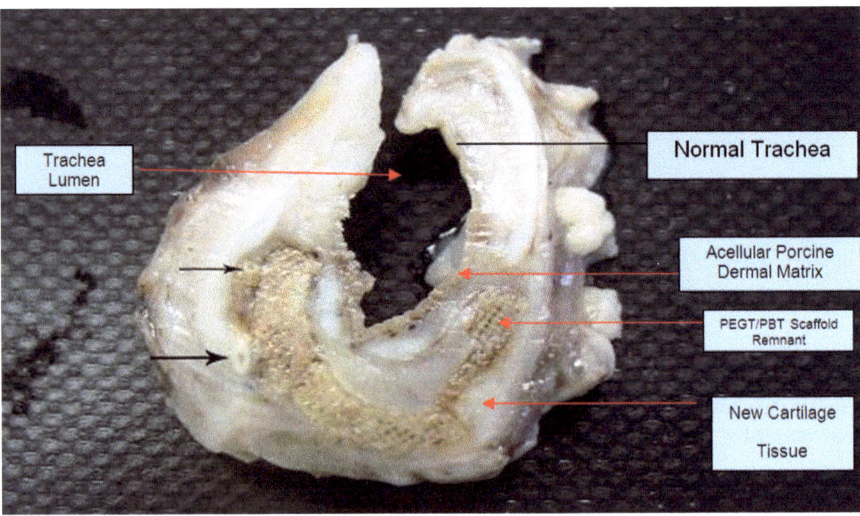

Fig. 5.13 Gross examination showed normal tracheal patency and cartilage tissue formation inside the PEGT/PBT scaffold

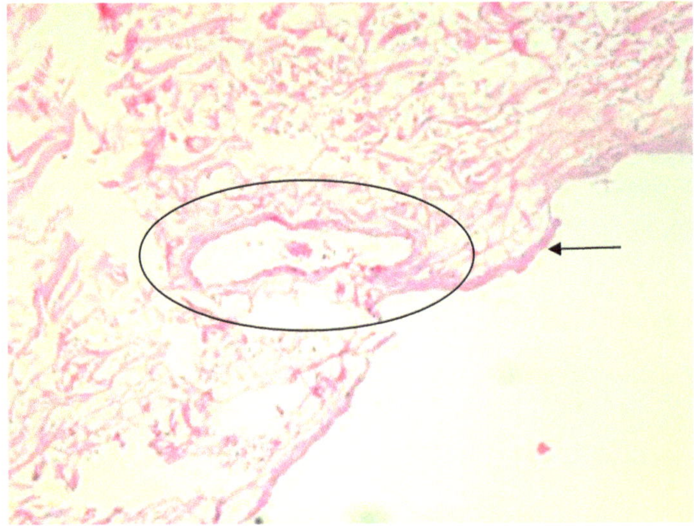

Fig. 5.14 Histology slides showed an intact epithelial layer (*black arrow*) on the surface of the acellular porcine dermal matrix and blood vessels inside (*black circle*)

Interestingly, the histology slides demonstrated an intact epithelial layer on the surface of the acellular porcine dermal matrix and vessel formation inside. Since we did not preseed the dermal matrix with any cells, these epithelial and endothelial cells definitely migrated from the normal tracheal tissue through the two anastomoses (Figs. 5.13, 5.14, and 5.15).

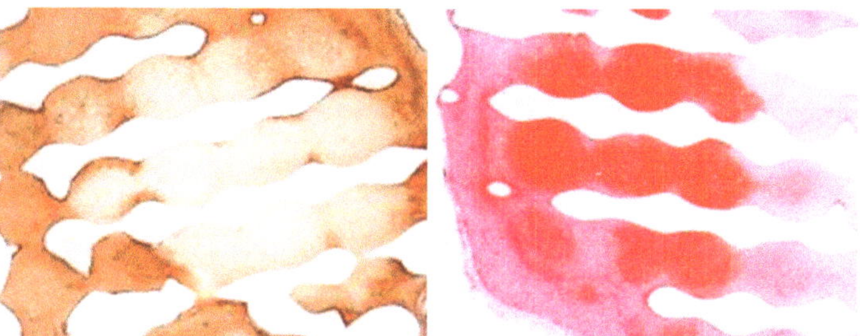

Fig. 5.15 Collagen II immunohistochemistry (*left*) and Safranin O staining (*right*) proved cartilage tissue formation

The sheep from the control group died 3 months after the operation. The autopsy showed tracheal lumen stenosis caused by granulation tissue overgrowth at the anastomosis site. Histology slides demonstrated serious contamination inside the patch where no cartilage tissue was found.

These results proved the feasibility of the in vivo bioreactor design in clinical applications using the standard process and equipment. The continuous perfusion with perfusate containing antibiotics, like pleural lavage for empyema treatment, reduced the possibility of contamination that stimulated granulation tissue overgrowth. The perfusion also accelerated reepithelialization and revascularization without preseeded cells. Studies using longer (4–6 cm) circumferential tracheal replacements and marked preseeded cells are required to further prove the advantages of the in vivo bioreactor design for TE trachea construction.

The Future

The regenerative capacity of human beings decreases with age-related consumption of stem cells and deterioration of the regenerative niche. Regenerative medicine aimed at reestablishing this power with cells, growth factors, and 3D scaffolds, individually and in combination with each other. Tissue engineering, a 3D cell culture technique that encompassed all three elements, represented the state of the art of regenerative medicine [54]. Limited knowledge of the regenerative niche and delayed angiogenesis after implantation frustrated the in vitro reconstruction and in vivo integration of traditional TE prostheses. The in vivo bioreactor design provides the opportunity to solve this problem through a survey of the natural regenerative niche. For example, a bone regeneration model was established by resection of 2 cm of a sheep rib while preserving the periosteum. Acellular porcine cancellous bone matrix was used as a bridge scaffold and a two-lumen perfusion catheter was placed over the matrix before periosteum closure. Continuous, closed-loop perfusion of

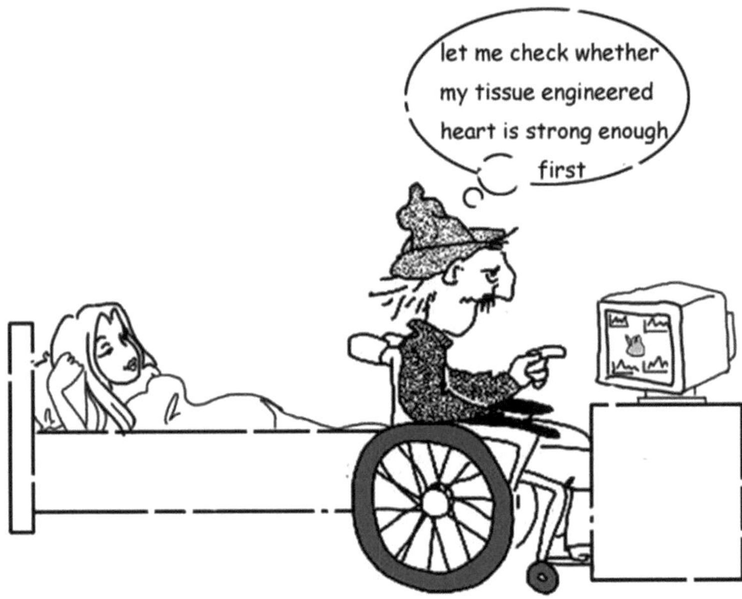

Fig. 5.16 "In-vivo bioreactor" combines with implantable biosensors might make monitoring and control of the tissue engineered organ regeneration process feasible

normal saline was established using two portable pumps. The perfusate was sampled every day for around 3 months until a bonelike high-density signal was detected by computed tomography scan. After bone regeneration was further proven through histological assessment, the concentration of growth factors associated with bone formation, such as bone morphologenetic protein (BMP), was measured in all of the collected samples to form a map of their spatial and temporal relationships during natural bone regeneration. Mass spectrometry of the perfusate samples might reveal some unknown proteins crucial to bone regeneration. The value of these data could be further validated in an in vitro bone regeneration bioreactor. It could also provide information to guide expansion of bone marrow stromal cells in vitro, as well as their induction into osteoblasts. Since it is feasible to quickly and precisely control various growth factor concentrations in the in vivo bioreactor, it might be possible to reconstruct large, clinically relevant bone using a spatial and temporal relationship map of the normal bone regenerative niche obtained from the bone regeneration model. With the help of implanted biosensors and wireless data transmission, the regenerative process associated with TE prostheses could be monitored in real time and deviations corrected in a timely manner through the adjustment of proper growth factor concentrations in the perfusate (Fig. 5.16). It would be more practical to stimulate the recipients' own regenerative power through the supply of adequate cells, properly shaped 3D scaffolds, and the regenerative niche than to reconstruct a tissue or organ substitute entirely in vitro.

Additionally, information on normal tissue regeneration would also benefit oncology research. The tumor stem cell theory assumes tumors originate in an altered regenerative niche, which induces the expression of several oncogenes or suppressed antioncogene expression [55, 56]. Changes in regeneration patterns might be used as a biomarker for early diagnosis of cancer. In addition, research into potential antitumor therapies has involved blocking tumor angiogenesis, which directly opposes angiogenesis-related research for tissue engineering [57]. Knowledge of normal stem cell differentiation and normal angiogenesis from in vivo bioreactor analysis might provide several potential targets for novel therapies.

The human body is a renewable closed system with a critical capacity to recognize self and nonself. Artificial organ prostheses often isolated from this system by fibrous encapsulation and allogeneic transplant rejection might manage to integrate by compromising the immune system [58–60]. However, this makes the recipient susceptible to infection and tumor formation. Tissue engineering aims to strengthen the regenerative capacity of this system by supplying vitality (cells), shape (3D scaffold), and the appropriate regenerative niche (various growth factors). The in vivo bioreactor presents an efficient way to combine these three basic elements and provides us with a tool to explore the natural regenerative process. Integrating it with biosensors could make it possible to monitor and further adjust the regenerative process associated with TE prostheses in situ and in real time.

References

1. Langer R, Vacanti JP. Tissue engineering. Science 1993;260:920–6.
2. Cao Y, Vacanti JP, Paige KT, Upton J, Vacanti CA. Transplantation of chondrocytes utilizing a polymer-cell construct to produce tissue-engineered cartilage in the shape of a human ear. Plast Reconstr Surg. 1997 Aug;100(2):297–302
3. Miller JS, Stevens KR, Yang MT, Baker BM, Nguyen DH, Cohen DM, Toro E, Chen AA, Galie PA, Yu X, Chaturvedi R, Bhatia SN, Chen CS. Rapid casting of patterned vascular networks for perfusable engineered three-dimensional tissue. Nat Mater. 2012 Jul 1(Epub ahead of print).
4. Lovett M, Lee K, Edwards A, Kaplan DL. Vascularization strategies for tissue engineering. Tissue Eng Part B Rev. 2009 Sep;15(3):353–70.
5. Visconti RP, Kasyanov V, Gentile C, Zhang J, Markwald RR, Mironov V. Towards organ printing: engineering an intra-organ branched vascular tree. Expert Opin Biol Ther. 2010 Mar;10(3):409–20.
6. Novosel EC, Kleinhans C, Kluger PJ. Vascularization is the key challenge in tissue engineering. Adv Drug Deliv Rev. 2011 Apr 30;63(4–5):300–11.
7. Jungebluth P, Bader A, Baiquera S, Moeller S, Jaus M, Lim ML, Fried K, Kjartansdottir KR, Go T, Nave H, Harringer W, Lundin V, Teixeira AI, Macchiarini P. The concept of in vivo airway tissue engineering. Biomaterials. 2012 Jun;33(17):4319–26.
8. Umeda H, Kanemaru S, Yamashita M, Ohno T, Suehiro A, Tamura Y, Hirano S, Nakamura T, Omori K, Ito J. In situ tissue engineering of canine skull with guided bone regeneration. Acta Otolaryngol. 2009 Dec;129(12):1509–18.
9. Groeber F, Holeiter M, Hampel M, Hinderer S, Schenke-Layland K. Skin tissue engineering – in vivo and in vitro applications. Adv Drug Deliv Rev. 2011 Apr 30;63(4–5):352–66.
10. Kock L, van Donkelaar CC, Ito K. Tissue engineering of functional articular cartilage: the current status. Cell Tissue Res. 2012 Mar; 347(3):613–27.

11. Rauh J, Milan F, Guenther KP, Stiehler M. Bioreactor systems for bone tissue engineering. Tissue Eng Part B Rev. 2011 Aug;17(4):263–80.
12. Kehoe DE, Jing D, Lock LT, Tzanakakis ES. Scalable stirred-suspension bioreactor culture of human pluripotent stem cells. Tissue Eng Part A. 2010 Feb;16(2):405–21.
13. Tan GK, Dinnes DL, Myers PT, Cooper-White JJ. Effects of biomimetic surfaces and oxygen tension on redifferentiation of passaged human fibrochondrocytes in 2D and 3D cultures. Biomaterials. 2011 Aug;32(24):5600–14.
14. Hoshiba T, Yamada T, Lu H, Kawazoe N, Chen G. Maintenance of cartilaginous gene expression on extracellular matrix derived from serially passaged chondrocytes during in vitro chondrocyte expansion. J Biomed Mater Res A. 2012 Mar;100(3):694–702.
15. Nguyen LH, Annabi N, Nikkhah M, Bae H, Binan L, Park S, Kang Y, Yang Y, Khademhosseini A. Vascularized bone tissue engineering: approaches for potential improvement. Tissue Eng Part B Rev. 2012 Jul 6 (Epub ahead of print).
16. Weber AD, Pontiggia L, Biedemann T, Schiestl C, Meuli M, Reichmann E. Determining the origin of cells in tissue engineered skin substitutes: a pilot study employing in situ hybridization. Pediatr Surg Int. 2011 Mar;27(3):255–61.
17. Zani BG, Kojima K, Vacanti CA, Edelman ER. Tissue-engineered endothelial and epithelial implants differentially and synergistically regulate airway repair. Proc Natl Acad Sci USA. 2008 May 13;105(19):7046–51.
18. Lee K, Silvia EA, Mooney DJ. Growth factor delivery-based tissue engineering: general approaches and a review of recent developments. J R Soc Interface. 2011 Feb 6;8(55): 153–70.
19. Madonna R, De Caterina R. Stem cells and growth factor delivery systems for cardiovascular disease. J Biotechnol 2011 Jul 20;154(4):291–7.
20. Sood S, Gupta S, Mahendra A. Gene therapy with growth factors for periodontal tissue engineering- a review. Med Oral Patol Oral Cir Bucal 2012 Mar 1;17(2):301–10.
21. Werkmeister JA, Ramshaw JA. Recombinant protein scaffolds for tissue engineering. Biomed Mater. 2012 Feb;7(1):012002
22. Tan Q, Steiner R, Heostrup SP, Weder W. Tissue-engineered trachea: history, problems and the future. Eur J Cardiothorac Surg. 2006;30(5):782–6.
23. Tan Q, Steiner R, Yang L, Welti M, Neuenschwander P, Hillinger S, Weder W. Accelerated angiogensis by continuous medium flow with vascular endothelial growth factor inside tissue-engineered trachea. Eur J Cardiothorac Sur. 2007;31(5):806–11.
24. Baiguera S, D'Innocenzo B, Macchiarini P. Current status of regenerative replacement of the airway. Expert Rev Respir Med. 2011 Aug;5(4):487–94.
25. Grillo HC. The History of tracheal surgery. Chest Surg Clin N Am. 2003;13:175–89.
26. Belsey R. Resection and reconstruction of the intrathoracic trachea. Br J Surg. 1950;38: 200–205.
27. Saad B, Hirt TD, Welti M, Uhlschmid GK, Neuenschwander P, Suter UW. Development of degradable polyesterurethanes for medical applications: in vitro and in vivo evaluations. J Biomed Master Res. 1997;36:65–74.
28. Bettahalli NM, Vicente J, Moroni L, Higuera GA, van Blitterswijk CA, Wessling M, Stamatialis DF. Integration of hollow fiber membranes improves nutrient supply in three-dimensional tissue constructs. Acta Biomater. 2011 Sep;7(9):3312–24.
29. Radisic M, Deen W, Langer R, Vunjak-Novakovic G. Mathematical model of oxygen distribution in engineered cardiac tissue with parallel channel array perfused with culture medium containing oxygen carriers. Am J Physiol Heart Circ Physiol. 2005 Mar;288(3):H 1278–89.
30. Tan Q, El-Badry A, Contaldo C, Steiner R, Hillinger S, Welti M, Spahn D, Higuera G, van Blitterswjik C, Luo QQ, Weder W. The effect of perfluorocarbon-based artificial oxygen carriers on tissue-engineered trachea. Tissue Eng. 2009 Sep;15(9):2471–80.
31. Maillard E, Juszczak MT, Langlois A, Kleiss C, Sencier M, Bietiger W, Sanchez-Dominguez M, Krafft MP, Johnson PR, Pinget M, Sigrist S. Perfluorocarbon emulsions prevent hypoxia of pancreatic beta-cells. Cell Transplant. 2011 Sep 22.

32. Feng X, Shen R, Tan J, Chen X, Pan Y, Ruan S, Zhang F, Lin Z, Zeng Y, Wang X, Lin Y, Wu Q. Burns. 2007 Jun;33(4):477–9.
33. Moroni L, Hendriks JA, Schotel R, den Wijn JR, van Blitterswijk CA. Design of biphasic polymeric 3-dimensional fiber deposited scaffolds for cartilage tissue engineering applications. Tissue Eng. 2007 Feb;13(2):361–71.
34. Maddison L, Karjagin J, Tenhunen J, Starkopf J. Moderate intra-abdominal hypertension is associated with an increased lactate-pyryvate ratio in the rectus abdominis muscle tissue: a pilot study during laparoscopic surgery. Ann Intensive Care. 2012 Jul 5;2 Suppl 1:S14.
35. Dransfeld CL, Alborzinia H, Woelfl S, Mahlknecht U. Continuous multiparametric monitoring of cell metabolism in response to transient overexpression of the sirtuin deacetylase SIRT3. Clin Epigenetics. 2010 Sep;1(1–2):55–60.
36. Li X, Zhao L, Chen Z, Lin Y, Yu P, Mao L. Continuous electrochemical monitoring of extracellular lactate production from neonatal rat cardiomyocytes following myocardial hypoxia. Anal Chem. 2012 Jun 19;84(12):5285–91.
37. Ogata M, Awaji T, Twasaki N, Fujimaki R, Takizawa M, Maruyama K, Iwamoto Y, Uchigata Y. A new mitochondrial pH biosensor for quantitative assessment of pancreatic beta-cell function. Biochem Biophys Res Commun. 2012 Apr 27;421(1):20–6
38. Lokmic Z, Mitchell GM. Engineering the microcirculation. Tissue Eng Part B Rev. 2008 Mar;14(1):87–103.
39. Baiguera S, D'Innocenzo B, Macchiarini P. Current status of regenerative replacement of the airway. Expert Rev Respir Med. 2011 Aug;5(4):487–94.
40. Francioli SE, Candrian C, Martin K, Heberer M, Martin I, Barbero A. Effect of three-dimensional expansion and cell seeding density on the cartilage-forming capacity of human articular chondrocytes in type II collagen sponges. J Biomed Mater Res A. 2012 Dec 1;95(3):924–31.
41. Yeatts AB, Fisher JP. Tubular perfusion system for the long-term dynamic culture of human mesenchymal stem cells. Tissue Eng Part C Methods. 2011 Mar;17(3):337–48.
42. Krawetz R, Rancourt DE. Suspension bioreactor expansion of undifferentiated human embryonic stem cells. Methods Mol Biol. 2012;873:227–35.
43. Tan Q, HillingerS, van Blitterswijk CA, Weer W. Intra-scaffold continuous medium flow combines chondrocyte seeding and culture systems for tissue engineered trachea construction. Interact Cardiovasc Thorac Surg. 2009 Jan;8(1):27–30.
44. Olivares AL, Lacroix D. Simultation of cell seeding within a three-dimensional porous scaffold: a fluid-particle analysis. Tissue Eng Part C Methods. 2012 Aug;18(8):624–31.
45. Mohebbi-Kalhori D, Rukhlova M, Ajji A, Bureau M, Moreno MJ. A novel automated cell-seeding device for tissue engineering of tubular scaffolds: design and functional validation. J Tissue Eng Regen Med. 2011 Sep 22.
46. Melchels FP, Tonnarelli B, Olivares AL, Martin I, Lacroix D, Feijen J, Wendt DJ, Grijpma DW. The influence of the scaffold design on the distribution of adhering cells after perfusion cell seeding. Biomaterials. 2011 Apr;32(11):2878–84.
47. Yoon HH,Bhang SH, Shin JY, Shin J, Kim BS. Enchanced cartilage formation via three-dimensional cell engineering of human adipose-derived stem cells. Tissue Eng Part A. 2012 Aug 10.
48. Caron MM, Emans PJ, Coolsen MM, Voss L, Surtel DA, Cremers A, van Rhijn LW, Welting TJ. Redifferentiation of dedifferenciated human articular chondrocytes: comparison of 2D and 3D cultures. Osteoarthritis Cartilage. 2012 Jul 10.
49. Iwata K, Asawa Y, Nishizawa S, Mori Y, Nagata S, Takato T, Hoshi K. The development of a serum-free medium utilizing the interaction between growth factors and biomaterials. Biomaterials. 2012 Jan;33(2):444–54.
50. Janicki P, Schmidmaier G. What should be the characteristics of the ideal bone graft substitute? Combining scaffolds with growth factors and/or stem cells. Injury. 2011 Sep;42 Suppl 2: S77-81.
51. Chu H, Wang Y. Therapeutic angiogenesis: controlled delivery of angiogenic factors. Ther Deliv. 2012 Jun;3(6):693–714.

52. Macchiarini P, Jungebluth P, Go T, Asnaghi MA, Rees LE, Cogan TA, Dodson A, Martorell J, Bellini S, Parnigotto PP, Dickinson SC, Hollander AP, Mantero S, Conconi MT, Birchall MA. Clinical transplantation of a tissue-engineered airway. Lancet. 2008 Dec 13;372(9655): 2023–30.
53. Jungebluth P, Baser A, Baiguera S, Moeller S, Jaus M, Lim ML, Fried K, Kjatansdottir KR, Go T, Nave H, Harringer W, Lundin V, Teixeira AI, Macchiarini P. The concept of in vivo airway tissue engineering. Biomaterials. 2012 Jun;33(17):4319–26.
54. Couto DS, Perez-Breva L, Cooney CL. Regenerative medicine: learning from past examples. Tissue Eng Part A. 2012 Jul 25.
55. Gilbertson RJ, Graham TA. Cancer: resolving the stem-cell debate. Nature. 2012 Aug 1
56. Bailey AM. Balancing tissue and tumor formation in regenerative medicine. Sci Transl Med. 2012 Aug 15;4(147):147fs28.
57. Shojaei F. Anti-angiogenesis therapy in cancer: current challenges and future perspectives. Cancer Lett. 2012 Jul 28;320(2):130–7.
58. Bryers JD, Giachelli CM, Ratner BD. Engineering biomaterials to integrate and heal: the biocompatibility paradigm shifts. Biotechnol Bioeng. 2012 Aug;109(8):1898–911.
59. Brown BN, Ratner BD, Goodman SB, Amar S, Badylak SF. Macrophage polarization: an opportunity for improved outcomes in biomaterials and regenerative medcine. Biomaterials. 2012 May;33(15):3792–802.
60. Franz S, Rammelt S, Scharnweber D, Simon JC. Immune responses to implants- a review of the implications for the design of immunomodulatory biomaterials. Biomaterials. 2011 Oct;32(28):6692–709.

Part II

Chapter 6
Segue

Wayne Burleson and Sandro Carrara

The book takes a significant turn at this point, moving from Part I, which involves the design of novel biosensors, to Part II, which shows the design of secure implantable medical devices. Key threads that cross between the two sections (Fig. 6.1) are:

- What data are produced (size, rate, resolution, statistics)?
- What value do those data have? In isolation? Or when combined with other data? How are the data used?
- What vulnerabilities arise in the sensor architecture? Can data be modified? Viewed by unauthorized parties? Can the origin and integrity of the data be assured?
- What conditions must be maintained in order to ensure proper acquisition of data (voltage, temperature, time, sampling)?
- What actuators are used in IMD systems and what vulnerabilities do they introduce? Can electrical therapies and drug delivery systems result in fatal outcomes?
- What intellectual property is contained in IMDs that can be stolen or violated through counterfeiting?

The book's last two chapters on security also extend beyond the case of sensors to devices; these include actuators that are essential, especially in cases such as implantable bioreactors. This also includes drug delivery systems and systems that deliver electrotherapies such as pacing and defibrillation for cardiology or electrostimulation for pain relief.

W. Burleson (✉)
Department of Electrical and Computer Engineering, University of Massachusetts,
309C Knowles Engineering Building, Amherst 01003, USA
e-mail: Burleson@ecs.umass.edu

S. Carrara
École polytechnique fédérale de Lausanne, Lausanne, Switzerland
e-mail: Sandro.carrara@epfl.ch

W. Burleson and S. Carrara (eds.), *Security and Privacy for Implantable Medical Devices*, DOI 10.1007/978-1-4614-1674-6_6,

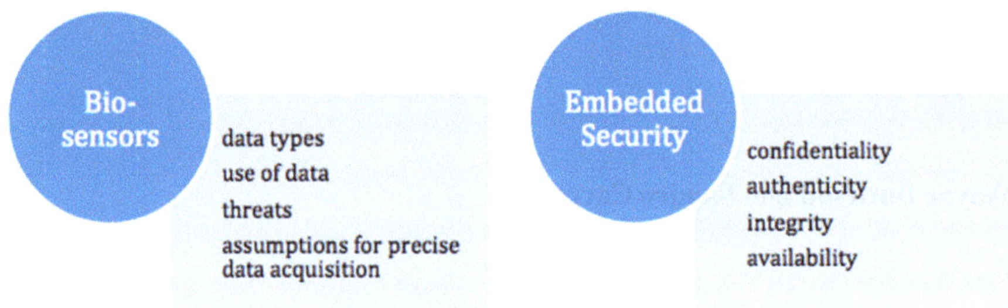

Fig. 6.1 Connections in the two fields of biosensors and security devices

Another area that is treated in this part is the eventual use of data and additional vulnerabilities that may be introduced at higher levels.

Chapter 7
Design Challenges for Secure Implantable Medical Devices

Benjamin Ransford, Shane S. Clark, Denis Foo Kune, Kevin Fu, and Wayne P. Burleson

Introduction

Implantable medical devices (IMDs) perform a variety of therapeutic or life-saving functions ranging from drug infusion and cardiac pacing to direct neurostimulation. They improve patients' quality of life by providing constant care.

Modern IMDs are electronic devices with hardware and software on board. They use low-power components to perform sensing, computation, and actuation, in some cases without patient involvement. Many include wireless clinical interfaces to support data collection and therapy adjustments.

Because of their crucial roles in patient health, IMDs undergo rigorous evaluation to verify that they meet regulatory requirements. Regulators such as the U.S. Food and Drug Administration (FDA) are required to evaluate products for *safety* and *effectiveness*, and manufacturers' processes are commonly geared toward meeting these specific goals. *Security* is a relatively new—but crucial—regulatory concern.

B. Ransford (✉)
Computer Science and Engineering, University of Washington
e-mail: ransford@cs.washington.edu

S.S. Clark
School of Computer Science, University of Massachusetts Amherst
e-mail: ssclark@cs.umass.edu

D.F. Kune • K. Fu
Computer Science and Engineering, University of Michigan
e-mail: dfkune@umich.edu; kevinfu@umich.edu

W.P. Burleson
Department of Electrical and Computer Engineering, University of Massachusetts,
309C Knowles Engineering Building, Amherst, MA 01003, USA
e-mail: Burleson@ecs.umass.edu

W. Burleson and S. Carrara (eds.), *Security and Privacy for Implantable Medical Devices*, 157
DOI 10.1007/978-1-4614-1674-6_7, © Springer Science+Business Media New York 2014

A system's security properties are a major determinant of the system's overall trustworthiness [16]. Poor security can severely affect other aspects of trustworthiness such as reliability and safety. As IMDs evolve with more-complex software and come to resemble general-purpose computers in their capabilities, they face some of the same security risks as general-purpose computers.

Security problems in IMDs are not merely theoretical; they often emerge as unintended consequences when systems are enhanced in other ways. For example, when a cardiac implant gains a wireless interface for clinical monitoring, it may also expose the patient to malicious eavesdropping (a violation of privacy) or tampering [23]. Other risks include forced battery depletion [23] and the tracking of unwitting patients [44].

This chapter summarizes research demonstrating that some IMDs fail to meet appropriate expectations of security for critically important systems. The key classes of IMD vulnerabilities researchers have identified are *control* vulnerabilities, in which an unauthorized person can gain control of an IMD's operation or even disable its therapeutic services, and *privacy* vulnerabilities, in which an IMD exposes patient data to an unauthorized party. Both kinds of vulnerability may be harmful to patients' health outcomes, and both kinds are avoidable.

This chapter's goals are to (1) outline design principles for IMD security; (2) highlight the security challenges in designing implantable medical devices, some of which remain open problems; and (3) sketch the defensive measures that researchers have proposed and implemented.

Security Principles for IMD Design

The term *security* refers to the goal of well-defined, correct system behavior in the presence of adversaries.[1] Security is related to another design goal, reliability, in that both define policies and actions under adverse conditions. Together, security and reliability form the basis of *trustworthiness* [16].

Designers of IMDs should consider security in all design phases. To maintain an appropriate level of attention to security, it is helpful to revisit several rules of thumb continually throughout the design process. Later on, this chapter will explain each of these in detail.

1. **Build security in**. (Section "Software Development Practices") Do not try to "bolt on" security measures as an afterthought; doing so will result in unforeseen failure modes.
2. **Keep security mechanisms simple**. (Section "Software Development Practices") Simple systems make it easier to reason about security—and find vulnerabilities before an adversary does.
3. **Use standard tools**. (Section "Software Development Practices") Use industry-standard source-code analysis techniques at design time.

[1] See Bishop's textbook [6] for a comprehensive introduction to security.

4. **Obscurity does not provide security**. (Section "Using Cryptography") Assume an adversary can discover source code and design documents.
5. **Encrypt sensitive traffic**. (Section "Using Cryptography") If the IMD transmits sensitive data, encrypt the data to protect them from eavesdroppers.
6. **Use well-studied cryptographic building blocks**. (Section "Using Cryptography") If you are using cryptography, do not design your own ciphers or encryption schemes; use standard ciphers and protect the secret keys.
7. **Authenticate third-party devices**. (Section "Using Cryptography") Make external devices cryptographically prove that they are what they claim to be.
8. **Develop a realistic threat model**. (Section "Threat Modeling") Defend the most attractive targets—considering the value and ease of compromise of each—first.

These design principles are not specific to IMDs; they are fundamental security ideas. Applying them to the IMD domain requires special consideration of IMDs' use cases and limitations. For example, the choice of cryptographic system to implement on a tiny biosensor or nonrechargeable heart device can have major implications for battery longevity.

Halperin et al. detail some holistic design considerations related to medical-device security [22]. In contrast, this chapter focuses on device-level concepts, relating the foregoing principles to three specific classes of IMD (Section "Devices in Depth").

Software Development Practices

Security engineering is a key component of modern product design, especially as devices integrate more and more layers of complexity, each of which brings new potential vulnerabilities. The books by Anderson [1], Viega and McGraw [49], and McGraw [33] are practical introductions to sound security practices.

Companies may find it instructive to measure the success of their own security initiatives and compare them to those of other companies. The Building Security In Maturity Model (BSIMM) [34] is a descriptive study of software-security practices at 51 major companies. The key message of the BSIMM is that attention to security is necessary *at every stage* of product development—i.e., it must be "built in" to both products and companies. As a complement to technical security guides, the BSIMM discusses effective organizational structures (i.e., engineering roles and management positions) that minimize the chances of security flaws falling through the cracks. Designers should avail themselves of the tools and techniques these companies use to analyze and test their designs for security problems.

An aspect of all good security design is simplicity. In the words of the French writer Antoine de Saint-Exupéry, "It seems that perfection is attained not when there is nothing more to add, but when there is nothing more to remove." [9] Security problems creep in when it becomes too difficult for any one person to diagram. An example of runaway complexity materially affecting security is the 700-page specification for a European bank-card system; researchers discovered a simple, difficult-to-detect attack that was possible when they coaxed the components into a certain combination of operating states [36]. Attackers often seek "out-of-spec" configurations that designers may have failed to address. The best way to mitigate these risks is to keep the specifications simple.

Using Cryptography

Judicious use of cryptography is key to the design and deployment of devices that store or transmit sensitive data. The goals of data encryption and device authorization are relatively well defined, but choosing appropriate ciphers, cipher modes, and authentication protocols is not a straightforward task. In this section, we offer guidelines to avoid a number of common security design pitfalls. Ferguson et al. discuss these and related principles in more detail [14].

A fundamental tenet of cryptography, commonly known as Kerckhoffs' principle [29], is that a cryptosystem should be secure even if the adversary knows everything about the system except its key. Put another way, a designer should not rely on the *obscurity* of cryptographic mechanisms because obscurity is easy to defeat. A major implication of this rule is that system designers should choose well-understood, publicly studied cryptosystems instead of designing their own. By choosing a cryptosystem that has withstood public scrutiny by professional cryptographers, designers can rely on the expertise of an entire community.

A recent example that illustrates the hazards of "security through obscurity" is that of the NXP Mifare Classic smart-card chipset, used for ticketing in public transit systems worldwide. Nohl et al. *mechanically* reverse-engineered Mifare Classic chips in a laboratory to analyze the underlying cipher and protocol. They discovered that the Mifare Classic used a flawed implementation of a proprietary cipher called Crypto-1 [37] that supported only small key sizes, making the system susceptible to brute-force attacks. Additionally, the card's hardware implemented a predictable pseudorandom-number generator, resulting in the system's staying compromised once compromised. These factors combined to allow an adversary to clone a tag—perhaps for sale or fare stealing—in a matter of seconds. The Mifare Classic tag could have addressed these flaws by using established, publicly studied cryptographic primitives rather than ad hoc proprietary systems.

After choosing primitives, designers must apply those primitives appropriately to protect the sensitive data aggregated and sometimes transmitted by medical devices. Concrete implementation advice is available from Ferguson et al. [14] and Anderson [1]. Lenstra provides suggestions for systematically choosing key lengths for a variety of cryptosystems [31]. Failing to encrypt traffic or authenticate third-party devices can lead to major security problems, including leakage of private information or an attacker who gains control over a device. The sections "Insulin Pump: Open-Loop System" and "Defibrillator: Closed-Loop System" give specific examples of some of the compromises possible when devices do not encrypt or authenticate information.

Threat Modeling

Threat modeling, which entails anticipating and characterizing potential threats, is a vital aspect of security design. With realistic models of adversaries, designers can assign appropriate priorities to addressing different threats.

The severity of vulnerabilities varies along with the sensitivity of the data or the consequences of actuation; there is no one-size-fits-all threat model for IMDs. A nonactuating glucose sensor incurs different risks than a defibrillator that can deliver disruptive electrical shocks to a heart.

Adversaries are typically characterized by their goals, their capabilities, and the resources they possess. Security designers evaluate each threat by considering the value of the target and the amount of effort necessary to access it. Recent work analyzing IMD security and privacy has posited several classes of adversaries, described below.

An *eavesdropper* who listens to an IMD's radio transmissions, but does not interfere with them, can often learn private information with minimal effort. Such a *passive adversary* may have access to an oscilloscope, software radio, directional antennas, and other listening equipment. Several studies have considered this type of adversary and demonstrated that eavesdropping on unencrypted communications could compromise patient data privacy [24, 32, 39, 42, 44].

An *active adversary* extends the passive adversary's capabilities with the ability to generate radio transmissions addressed to the IMD or to replay recorded control commands. Halperin et al. demonstrated that an active adversary with a programmable radio could control one model of implantable defibrillator by replaying messages—disabling programmed therapies or even delivering a shock intended to induce a fatal heart rhythm [24]. Jack and Li have demonstrated similar control over an insulin pump, including the ability to stop insulin delivery or inject excessive doses [32, 44].

Active adversaries may also attempt to manipulate the inputs to the system in an effort to affect the output. The input leads of IMDs measure potential differences and may be vulnerable to signal injection using electromagnetic interference (EMI) [15]. If allowed to reach the sensing inputs, EMI signals may alter pacing or defibrillation therapy delivery, although the reported range in human phantoms is limited.

Another adversarial capability is *binary analysis*, the ability to disassemble a system's software and in some cases completely understand its operation. By inspecting the Java-based configuration program supplied with his own insulin pump, researcher Jerome Radcliffe reverse-engineered the pump's packet structure, revealing that the pump failed to encrypt the medical data it transmitted or to adequately authenticate the components to one another [42]. In contrast to design-time static analysis of source code, a crucial practice that may expose flaws before devices are shipped [28], binary analysis involves inspecting *compiled* code; it can expose flaws in systems that erroneously depend on the supposed difficulty of reverse engineering to conceal private information.

In the context of medical conditions, it may be difficult to comprehend why a malicious person would seek to cause harm to patients receiving therapy, but unfortunately, it has happened in the past. For example, in 2008, malicious hackers defaced a Web page run by the nonprofit Epilepsy Foundation, replacing the page's content with flashing animations that induced migraines or seizures for some unsuspecting visitors [40]. Although we know of no reports of malicious attacks against IMDs "in the wild," it is important to address vulnerabilities before they become serious threats.

Finally, to complement the guides to software security mentioned in previous sections, designers should familiarize themselves with attack techniques. A good start is a book by Hoglund and McGraw [26]. Good adversaries, however, move too fast to capture between book covers; popular online resources such as the Common Vulnerabilities and Exposures database [35] are constantly updated as attacks and defenses evolve.

Policy Planning

Beyond threat modeling and the adoption of publicly studied security primitives, IMD designers must also consider security policies. While security policy may seem like an issue outside the purview of device designers, long product lifecycles and restrictive regulatory environments elevate policy to design-time problem for IMDs—particularly those that incorporate or interact with commodity operating systems or software. IMDs successfully complete validation only once before release to market, and software changes after validation potentially carry legal and reliability ramifications. Despite these ramifications, device designers and manufacturers have a responsibility to plan for changes in response to vulnerability discoveries.

Some implantable cardiac defibrillator (ICD) designers already address the problem of software updates. Gaining physical access to a fully implanted device like an ICD is a potential health risk, so wireless software updates performed in a clinical setting are an established practice. The difficult questions to address in the general case are when and where software updates are appropriate and necessary. Patient safety is the highest priority. As such, the rapid delivery of safety or reliability updates is an important goal, but allowing updates in unconstrained or poorly verified environments can pose both safety and security risks that must be balanced with rapid and widespread deployment.

Another important consideration when formulating policies is the regulatory environment in which devices will operate over the course of their market lifetimes. In the United States, the FDA sets standards for device updates through the 510(k) process [47]. Significant updates to devices already on the market require new clearance or a declaration of *substantial equivalence* to an existing device before being released to market. A tempting conclusion for manufacturers is that the liabilities and complications inherent in this process justify a "no security updates" stance [4], but FDA guidance on the issue in fact specifically states that device owners should "update [their] operating system and medical device software" [48].

One step toward addressing policy issues proactively at design time is to apply the outputs of threat modeling not just to initial device design but to mitigation strategies in the event that vulnerabilities are discovered. Knowing where the possible points of access are for an adversary and understanding the steps necessary to address different vulnerability scenarios can inform the design process through a feedback process. Designers can also advocate for clear statements and policies regarding security issues at the company level because threat modeling gives them a unique perspective on future complications.

Devices in Depth

To illustrate the complexity of the design space for IMD security, we offer three examples of IMD systems that pose different security challenges because of their different design and usage. The common thread among all three devices—insulin pump systems, implantable cardiac defibrillators, and subcutaneous biosensors—is that security is a crucial design concern. The section "Common Threads" explores commonalities and defensive concepts.

Insulin Pump: Open-Loop System

Insulin pump systems (IPSs) straddle the boundary between implanted and external systems, including some components that are physically attached to a patient and others that are external. A typical modern IPS may include an insulin infusion pump with wireless interface that subcutaneously delivers insulin, a continuous glucose monitor (CGM) with wireless transmitter and subcutaneous sensor for glucose measurement, and a wireless remote control that the patient can use to alter infusion pump settings or manually trigger insulin injections. CGMs automatically take frequent glucose readings, presenting the data to the user via a screen or PC, or sending data directly to the pump. The pump automatically provides *basal* doses for insulin maintenance and can also administer larger *bolus* doses to compensate for large insulin spikes that may result from, for example, a meal. Finally, the remote control provides a convenient interface for the user to adjust pump settings without using the pump controls and screen typically attached at the abdomen. Figure 7.1 shows a block diagram of an IPS.

IPSs exemplify *open-loop* IMDs: they require patient interaction to change pump settings. Specifically, the patient's remote control—but not the CGM—directly controls pump actuation. Because the remote-control interface carries crucial information and control signals, initial security studies have focused on finding vulnerabilities at this interface. Li et al. discovered that one IPS's communications were unencrypted, leading to potential disclosure of private patient information (e.g., glucose levels) [32]. They also found that the components failed to check their inputs

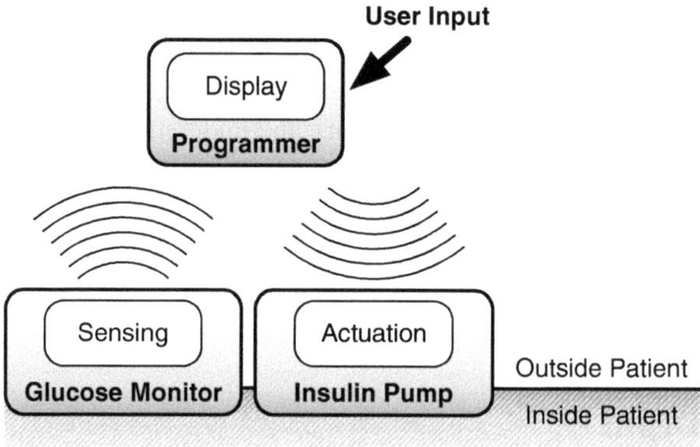

Fig. 7.1 Block diagram of an insulin pump system (IPS), an open-loop IMD

appropriately, allowing the researchers to inject forged packets reporting incorrect glucose levels to the patient and pump— and, more alarmingly, to issue unauthorized pump-control commands. Soon thereafter, two security researchers independently demonstrated full control of IPSs via the circumvention of authentication mechanisms: Radcliffe compromised the wireless channel of his own (unspecified) IPS [42, 46], and Jack performed a live demonstration in which he remotely controlled and then shut down a volunteer's insulin pump [44]. Jack also demonstrated that certain IPSs responded to anonymous radio scanning with their serial numbers, a privacy vulnerability because of the potential of tracking IPS patients.

Challenges of open-loop systems. Because open-loop systems incorporate users into the control loop, the users themselves are an important part of the device attack surface. Threats to open-loop systems that target the user are the focus of an entire subfield of security termed *usable security*. An adversary need not completely compromise a device if she can instead fool a user into making unsafe adjustments. In the case of an IPS, an adversary could alter the glucose reading shown to a user, leading the user to inject too much or too little insulin, for example. Any user interface where a human must interpret outputs or provide inputs provides a potential entry point for such malicious tampering.

Much of the abundant research on usable security seeks to address the issue of secure user interface design [7, 45], which is a key concern for medical devices operated by patients, who are not likely to have expert knowledge of the specific devices they use. Providing users with unambiguous indications of their device's state and the tools to make informed security decisions are key goals that require careful consideration. The work of Sunshine et al. [45] underscores how difficult it can be to alter user behavior, even in the presence of what a designer might consider to be clear warning signs. Secure interface design requires the designer to understand that users will not necessarily maintain a security mindset.

Another major goal in the area of usable security is to ensure that users understand the possible security risks of their devices and are comfortable with deployed security measures. Denning et al. conducted a user study highlighting some of the security interface design issues pertaining specifically to IMDs [10]. They presented multiple security mockups to patients with cardiac implants to gauge patient attitudes toward both IMD security in general and the specific protections proposed. While the majority of patients surveyed agreed that they were concerned about their personal privacy and physical safety, most of them disagreed that they were concerned about unauthorized changes to IMD behavior. Denning et al. also found that patients were concerned about the use of companion devices (such as wristbands) that could identify them as people with medical implants or that would serve as constant reminders of their conditions.

Defibrillator: Closed-Loop System

Like an artificial pacemaker, which continually issues small electrical pulses to heart muscle to maintain a healthy rhythm, an *implantable cardiac defibrillator* (ICD) is implanted under the skin near the clavicle. ICDs extend the capabilities of artificial pacemakers with the ability to issue large (tens of joules) shocks to "reset" an unsustainable heart rhythm (arrhythmia). Figure 7.2 shows a block diagram of an ICD.

Unlike an insulin pump that accepts patient input via a user interface, a fully implanted device such as an ICD is a *closed-loop* system: under normal circumstances, its sensing function alone dictates its actuation activities. (Closed-loop IMDs typically also have special modes for in-clinic configuration and operation.) Halperin et al. enumerated the security and privacy challenges of closed-loop implanted systems in a 2008 article [22], focusing primarily on the tensions between security and utility.

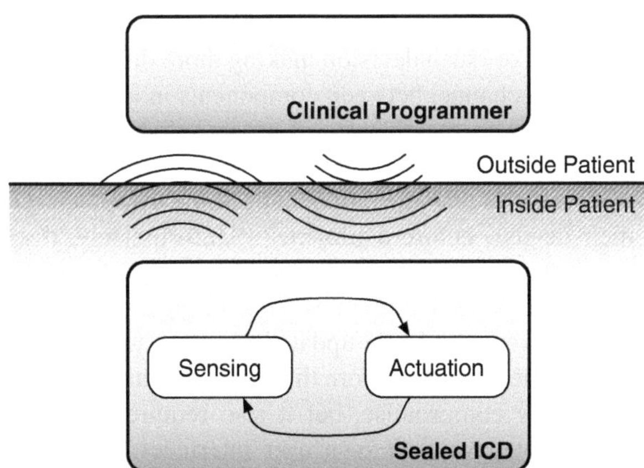

Fig. 7.2 Block diagram of an implantable cardiac defibrillator (ICD), a closed-loop IMD

ICD implantation currently requires invasive surgery with a risk of complications (infection or death) [19], so ICDs are designed to last for at least 5 years once implanted—resulting in long design and deployment cycles for manufacturers. ICDs draw power from single-use batteries, sealed inside the case, to provide uninterrupted monitoring throughout the device's lifetime and to avoid the heating of tissue that might occur during battery recharging. In conformance with these design choices, ICDs spend most of their time in low-power sensing states. They also include radios for clinical adjustments and at-home status reporting.

A 2008 security analysis of a commercial ICD found vulnerabilities in multiple subsystems [24], including those listed above. Focusing on the ICD's radio link, researchers used open-source software-radio tools to record transmissions between the ICD and a clinical programming console. Offline analysis of these traces revealed patient information in clear text without evidence of encryption. They replayed recorded traces of clinical therapy commands and found that they could control or disable the ICD's therapies with their software radio. Concerning the battery, the study found that a sequence of transmissions from the software radio could keep the ICD's radio in a high-power active mode, indefinitely transmitting packets at a regular rate and dramatically increasing the ICD's power consumption.

The radio interface is not the only vulnerable point; intentional EMI poses another risk. A 2013 paper describes analog signal injection of low-frequency waveforms (in the sub-30 kHz VLF range) on the sensing leads of IMDs, including ICDs [15]. With a carefully crafted EMI waveform and an implantable defibrillator with its leads in free air, the researchers confused the ICD's sensors and tricked the ICD into delivering a defibrillation shock. According to the paper, even an attacker who cannot perfectly match an EMI signal's wavelength to the length of the sensing leads can compensate by increasing the power of the EMI transmission, inducing millivolt-level signals at the IMD's sensing inputs.

Challenges of closed-loop systems. Compared to open-loop systems in which the user interface may be the weakest link, closed-loop systems are subject to different constraints. The key challenge for designers is to implement *automated* decision making as good as or better than an experienced clinician's. Modeling threats against a closed-loop system makes such decision making more difficult.

Establishing a secure channel between components in a closed-loop system can be a challenge, especially in the absence of a user interface. To authenticate one another, components generally must share a secret key, but there is no single best way to distribute secret keys among components. Some manufacturers predistribute secret keys to their devices before deployment. Unfortunately, if a predistributed secret key becomes compromised—for example, via hardware reverse engineering, the use of a weak cipher, or the incorrect use of a strong cipher—then every device with the compromised key should be updated. A more tractable alternative is to require customers to generate keys before they may use the devices. This approach limits the impact of key compromise, but it also requires a way to install keys on devices that may not have their own user interfaces. As another alternative, Halperin et al. offer a method of transcutaneous acoustic coupling for an ICD that

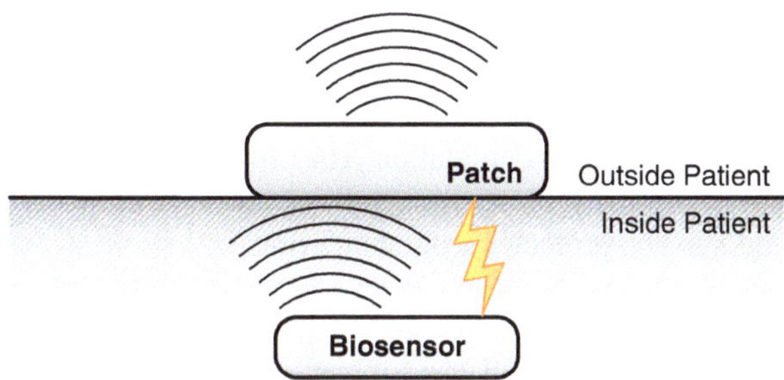

Fig. 7.3 Block diagram of a subcutaneous biosensor. Small biosensors may be injected into the patient and then inductively powered by a patch that relays sensed data to a higher-level wearable device

could be used to exchange key material [23]. Gollakota et al. propose a radio-based pairing mechanism that is *tamper evident* and works with devices that lack user interfaces [17].

Configuration without a user interface is another challenge that manufacturers have addressed in different ways. Critical parameters in closed-loop systems include configuration variables and actuation thresholds; reprogramming those variables could drastically alter the behavior of the system. Without a user interface allowing a continuous report on the status of the device, warning the user of a configuration change or a testing parameter in effect (e.g., a fibrillation test [23]) is difficult. Audio alerts (e.g., beeps) are common, but communicating to the user the reason for the alert and appropriate action can be challenging in this setting; patients may not respond favorably to voice prompts or beep warnings.

Finally, the output of a closed-loop system relies on the sensing inputs. An attacker controlling these inputs has some control over the system. Sensed time-dependent voltage levels, for example, may be vulnerable to analog signal injection via EMI as described earlier. In ICDs, the problem is even more acute because the mechanical constraints on the sensing leads prevent a true coaxial design—which is more prone to cracking—thereby making the leads more sensitive to EMI. Moreover, the devices need to sense in the subkilohertz band and therefore cannot use aggressive filtering in that range to combat EMI. In these systems, sanity checking at every component interface is critically important [15].

Biosensors for Data Acquisition

Implantable biosensors (Fig. 7.3) are IMDs that measure biological phenomena and send data to a more powerful device for storage or analysis. Biosensors are a broader device category than IPSs or defibrillators, representing a wide range of both signals and signal processing techniques. They are subject to a third set of security and privacy challenges that does not completely overlap with those mentioned earlier.

Biosensors range from high-data-rate imaging devices for the eye [5] or brain [41] to extremely low-data-rate sensors for glucose [20] or other metabolites in the blood [8]. Actuators that consume biosensor data can control potentially lethal drug-delivery systems [39] or electrical therapies [24]. Keeping biosensor data confidential is important because they can be used in illegal or unethical ways, including insurance fraud or discrimination. The provenance (origin) and timestamp information that accompany biosensor readings are also critically important for medical care and must be protected from tampering.

Subcutaneous biosensors present a special set of security and privacy requirements. A subcutaneous sensor [8] involves an implanted biosensor that acts as a *lab on a chip*, conducting a small experiment on the sensor at the molecular or electrochemical level. Current subcutaneous sensors can detect drugs, biomarkers, and antibodies and may eventually examine DNA and simultaneously log temperature, pH, and other phenomena.

Recent examples of subcutaneous biosensors include *injectable* subcutaneous devices that are remotely powered by a bandagelike patch that also provides a data link to a higher-level wearable device, possibly a body area network or, eventually, a higher-level health information system. A related class of devices are low-cost disposable biosensors for detecting infectious disease or critical levels of glucose and lactate in a battlefield or other trauma situation [21]; such devices penetrate the skin for communication and power. These two classes of devices support different threat models because of their different usage parameters.

Biosensors that are fully implanted must communicate wirelessly to transmit through tissue. (Some receive power through tissue as well; recent work has shown that remotely powering biosensors is feasible at gigahertz frequencies that enable millimeter-sized antennas [38].) A key problem with fully implanted sensors is that small, infrequent wireless transmissions may pose a greater privacy risk than large or continuous transmissions. For example, a sensor may take several minutes to complete its task, then deliver only a few bytes of data—giving this information a high value per bit that may make it an attractive target. Short data transmissions necessitate careful use of a cipher, especially if the plaintext sensor data take only a few different values. The small amount of data also has little inherent redundancy, making error correction necessary.

When a biosensor includes a patch that is meant to pair with the sensor, additional risks arise. Although eavesdropping on a properly operating tag may be unlikely because of the short (several millimeters for a subcutaneous sensor) nominal transmission range, impersonation of both the clinical reader and the patch are plausible concerns. For example, the patch of an unconscious patient can be removed and replaced by another patch. Similarly, a rogue sensor can upload fraudulent data to a trusted patch. All components involved should authenticate one another using well-studied cryptographic mechanisms, especially during the critically important period when a sensor is first being tested or calibrated.

Challenges of biosensor systems. Biosensors, with stringent space and energy constraints, present a diverse set of challenges for security and privacy. The limitations on energy and computational resources place many standard encryption primitives (such as ciphers and authentication schemes) out of reach, though advances in energy efficiency will likely expand the set of mechanisms that are practical. The main privacy risk arises from the unprecedented view into the inner workings of a patient's body; such information is presumably private and deserves protection.

New cryptosystems intended specifically for use on energy-constrained devices offer some hope for protecting user privacy on biosensors [12, 27], but the number of well-studied algorithms in this area is relatively small compared to the number of general-purpose cryptosystems.

Common Threads

Different classes of IMDs have distinct hardware and usage constraints, but there are important security considerations that apply to many IMDs. Researchers investigating the security and privacy of IMDs have also proposed several domain-specific mechanisms that apply broadly. This section discusses some of these common threads in the context of our example IMD systems.

All of the IMD communication vulnerabilities disclosed thus far could be mitigated by the use of appropriate cryptographic techniques on radio links. Hosseini-Khayat presents a lightweight wireless protocol for IMDs [27] that leverages well-studied wireless and cryptography technologies and emphasizes low-energy computation. The choice of encryption scheme should consider the nature of the data as well as the device constraints. Fan et al. contribute hardware implementations of the stream cipher Hummingbird [12, 13]. Beck explores the use of block ciphers in IMD security [5].

Unfortunately, cryptography is not a panacea for IMD security and privacy vulnerabilities; many questions remain. If the radio link were to use encryption, how would the necessary secret key material be distributed, and by whom? How should an IMD authenticate external entities, and how should it determine whether a particular entity is allowed to communicate with it? Even assuming that each of these questions can be answered, successful implementation of encryption would not completely address known risks. Encryption alone fails to address replay attacks, and previous work has demonstrated that encryption may not sufficiently conceal characteristic traffic patterns [25]. Furthermore, since some IMDs must "fail open" to allow emergency access (e.g., to disable the IMD during emergency procedures), how can they also provide security in non-emergency situations? Should an IMD raise an alarm (perhaps tactile or audible) when a security-sensitive event occurs? These questions are largely open.

Recent research aimed at addressing these design tensions has proposed new techniques and auxiliary devices to provide fail-open security for IMDs. Rasmussen et al. proposed the use of ultrasonic distance bounding to enforce programmer proximity [43]. Li et al. proposed body-coupled communications for the same purpose [32], hoping to prevent an adversary from launching a long-range, radio-based attack. Both of these distance-bounding techniques require new hardware, but this constraint may not represent a major stumbling block for IPSs or biosensor systems, which are short lived and noninvasive compared to ICDs.

Researchers have also proposed defenses that are specifically targeted toward existing ICDs but that may be useful for other IMDs. Denning et al. proposed that an IMD be paired with a *cloaker* that would provide authentication services whenever it was present, and allow open communication otherwise [11]. Xu et al. proposed the *Guardian*, a device that would pair with an IMD and use radio jamming to defend against eavesdropping and unauthorized commands [50]. Gollakota et al. independently proposed an auxiliary device called the *shield* that would use "friendly" radio jamming to proxy an ICD's communications to an authorized reader [18]. The shield is designed for compatibility with devices that are already implanted, reducing the burden on device designers to address the security vulnerabilities in devices that have not completed their deployment lifecycles.

Open Problems in IMD Design

IMDs are first and foremost intended to improve patients' quality of life. To this end, the primary focus for designers must be device safety and utility. We argue that security and privacy are also important properties that must be part of the design process, but there is the potential for direct conflict between these two sets of properties.

The issue of emergency access highlights some of the tensions that exist among these properties. Requiring users to authenticate to a device before altering its functionality is a boon for security, but it introduces risks in case of an emergency. A medical professional may need to reprogram or disable a device to effectively treat a patient. As discussed in the section "Common Threads," encryption or other strong authentication mechanisms could make such emergency measures impossible if the patient is unconscious or the facility does not possess a programming device with a required shared secret.

For some IMDs, including both IPSs and ICDs, designers must carefully weigh the energy costs of encryption against safety and utility. A heavyweight encryption scheme could potentially drain enough energy to require more frequent device replacement—a surgical procedure for ICD patients and a persistent burden for IPS users. Costly encryption could even make the construction and deployment of some subcutaneous biosensors infeasible. It remains to be seen whether ASIC implementations of lightweight algorithms can effectively mitigate this issue because of the lack of public deployments to date [5, 27].

There are no clear-cut methods for resolving these tensions, and there is little publicly available information about whatever steps manufacturers have already taken. While cryptographers and security researchers have long embraced Kerckhoffs' principle, device manufacturers employ proprietary systems and generally do not comment (for business reasons) on security measures that they may employ. These closed ecosystems hamper industrywide progress on shared issues such as security and privacy. Research into whole-system modeling and formal analysis of medical devices [2, 3, 30] offers hope that future IMDs will integrate sound security principles at design time, but the time horizon for industrial adoption may be long.

Recent analyses of implantable medical devices have revealed a number of security and privacy failings, but researchers are developing novel solutions to the problems IMD designers face. By incorporating security and privacy design principles into the development process, IMD designers have the opportunity to address these issues before they become larger threats.

Acknowledgements This material is based upon work supported by the Armstrong Fund for Science; the National Science Foundation (NSF) under Grants 831244, 0923313, and 0964641; Cooperative Agreement 90TR0003/01 from the Department of Health and Human Services (DHHS); two NSF Graduate Research Fellowships; and a Sloan Research Fellowship. Its contents are solely the responsibility of the authors and do not necessarily represent the official views of DHHS or NSF.

References

1. R. J. Anderson. *Security Engineering: A Guide to Building Dependable Distributed Systems.* Wiley, 2008.
2. D. Arney, R. Jetley, P. Jones, I. Lee, and O. Sokolsky. Formal methods based development of a PCA infusion pump reference model: Generic infusion pump (GIP) project. In *Proceedings of the 2007 Joint Workshop on High Confidence Medical Devices, Software, and Systems and Medical Device Plug-and-Play Interoperability*, HCMDSS-MDPNP '07, pages 23–33. IEEE Computer Society, 2007.
3. D. Arney, M. Pajic, J. M. Goldman, I. Lee, R. Mangharam, and O. Sokolsky. Toward patient safety in closed-loop medical device systems. In *Proceedings of the 1st ACM/IEEE International Conference on Cyber-Physical Systems*, ICCPS '10, pages 139–148. ACM, 2010.
4. Baxa Corporation. Preventing cyber attacks. https://btsp.baxa.com/Sales%20Portal/ExactaMix/Preventing%20Cyber%20Attacks.pdf, Loaded Oct. 2012.
5. C. Beck, D. Masny, W. Geiselmann, and G. Bretthauer. Block cipher based security for severely resource-constrained implantable medical devices. In *Proceedings of 4th International Symposium on Applied Sciences in Biomedical and Communication Technologies*, ISABEL '11, pages 62:1–62:5. ACM, October 2011.
6. M. Bishop. *Computer Security: Art and Science.* Addison-Wesley Professional, 2003.
7. S. Clark, T. Goodspeed, P. Metzger, Z. Wasserman, K. Xu, and M. Blaze. Why (special agent) johnny (still) can't encrypt: a security analysis of the apco project 25 two-way radio system. In *Proceedings of the 20th USENIX conference on Security.* USENIX Association, 2011.
8. G. De Micheli, S. Ghoreishizadeh, C. Boero, F. Valgimigli, and S. Carrara. An integrated platform for advanced diagnostics. In *Design, Automation & Test in Europe Conference & Exhibition*, DATE '11. IEEE, March 2011.
9. A. de Saint-Exupéry. *Terre des Hommes.* Editions Gallimard, 1939.
10. T. Denning, A. Borning, B. Friedman, B. T. Gill, T. Kohno, and W. H. Maisel. Patients, pacemakers, and implantable defibrillators: human values and security for wireless implantable medical devices. In *Proc. International Conference on Human Factors in Computing Systems (CHI)*, 2010.
11. T. Denning, K. Fu, and T. Kohno. Absence makes the heart grow fonder: New directions for implantable medical device security. In *Proceedings of USENIX Workshop on Hot Topics in Security (HotSec)*, July 2008.

12. X. Fan, G. Gong, K. Lauffenburger, and T. Hicks. FPGA implementations of the Hummingbird cryptographic algorithm. In *Proceedings of the IEEE International Symposium on Hardware-Oriented Security and Trust*, HOST '10, pages 48–51, June 2010.
13. X. Fan, H. Hu, G. Gong, E. Smith, and D. Engels. Lightweight implementation of Hummingbird cryptographic algorithm on 4-bit microcontrollers. In *International Conference for Internet Technology and Secured Transactions*, ICITST '09, pages 1–7, November 2009.
14. N. Ferguson, B. Schneier, and T. Kohno. *Cryptography Engineering: Design Principles and Practical Applications*. Wiley, 2010.
15. D. Foo Kune, J. Backes, S. S. Clark, D. B. Kramer, M. R. Reynolds, K. Fu, Y. Kim, and W. Xu. Ghost talk: mitigating EMI signal injection attacks against analog sensors. In *Proceedings of the 34th Annual IEEE Symposium on Security and Privacy*, May 2013.
16. K. Fu. Trustworthy medical device software. In *Public Health Effectiveness of the FDA 510(k) Clearance Process: Measuring Postmarket Performance and Other Select Topics: Workshop Report*, Washington, DC, July 2011. IOM (Institute of Medicine), National Academies Press.
17. S. Gollakota, N. Ahmed, N. Zeldovich, and D. Katabi. Secure in-band wireless pairing. In *Proceedings of the 20th USENIX Security Symposium*, August 2011.
18. S. Gollakota, H. Hassanieh, B. Ransford, D. Katabi, and K. Fu. They can hear your heartbeats: non-invasive security for implanted medical devices. In *Proceedings of ACM SIGCOMM*, Aug. 2011.
19. P. Gould and A. Krahn. Complications associated with implantable cardioverter–defibrillator replacement in response to device advisories. *Journal of the American Medical Association (JAMA)*, 295(16):1907–1911, April 2006.
20. S. Guan, J. Gu, Z. Shen, J. Wang, Y. Huang, and A. Mason. A wireless powered implantable bio-sensor tag system-on-chip for continuous glucose monitoring. In *Proceedings of the IEEE Biomedical Circuits and Systems Conference*, BioCAS '11, November 2011.
21. A. Guiseppi-Elie. An implantable biochip to influence patient outcomes following trauma-induced hemorrhage. *Analytical and Bioanalytical Chemistry*, 399(1):403–419, January 2011.
22. D. Halperin, T. S. Heydt-Benjamin, K. Fu, T. Kohno, and W. H. Maisel. Security and privacy for implantable medical devices. *IEEE Pervasive Computing, Special Issue on Implantable Electronics*, 7(1):30–39, January 2008.
23. D. Halperin, T. S. Heydt-Benjamin, B. Ransford, S. S. Clark, B. Defend, W. Morgan, K. Fu, T. Kohno, and W. H. Maisel. Pacemakers and implantable cardiac defibrillators: Software radio attacks and zero-power defenses. In *Proceedings of the 29th Annual IEEE Symposium on Security and Privacy*, pages 129–142, May 2008.
24. D. Halperin, T. S. Heydt-Benjamin, B. Ransford, S. S. Clark, B. Defend, W. Morgan, K. Fu, T. Kohno, and W. H. Maisel. Pacemakers and implantable cardiac defibrillators: Software radio attacks and zero-power defenses. In *Proceedings of the 29th IEEE Symposium on Security and Privacy*, May 2008.
25. A. Hintz. Fingerprinting websites using traffic analysis. In R. Dingledine and P. Syverson, editors, *Proceedings of the Privacy Enhancing Technologies workshop*, PET '02. Springer, LNCS 2482, April 2002.
26. G. Hoglund and G. McGraw. *Exploiting Software: How to Break Code*. Addison-Wesley Professional, 2004.
27. S. Hosseini-Khayat. A lightweight security protocol for ultra-low power ASIC implementation for wireless implantable medical devices. In *Proceedings of the 5th International Symposium on Medical Information Communication Technology*, ISMICT '11, pages 6–9, March 2011.
28. R. P. Jetley, P. L. Jones, and P. Anderson. Static analysis of medical device software using CodeSonar. In *Proceedings of the 2008 Workshop on Static Analysis*, SAW '08, pages 22–29. ACM, 2008.
29. A. Kerckhoffs. La cryptographie militaire. *Journal des Sciences Militaires*, IX, Jan 1883.
30. I. Lee, G. J. Pappas, R. Cleaveland, J. Hatcliff, and B. H. Krogh. High-confidence medical device software and systems. *IEEE Computer*, 39(4):33–38, 2006.
31. A. K. Lenstra. Key lengths. In H. Bidgoli, editor, *Handbook of Information Security, Volume 1: Key Concepts, Infrastructure, Standards and Protocols.*, page ... John Wiley, 2006.

32. C. Li, A. Raghunathan, and N. K. Jha. Hijacking an insulin pump: security attacks and defenses for a diabetes therapy system. In *Proceedings of the 13th IEEE International Conference on e-Health Networking, Applications, and Services*, Healthcom '11, June 2011.
33. G. McGraw. *Software Security: Building Security In*. Addison-Wesley Professional, 2006.
34. G. McGraw, S. Migues, and J. West. *Building Security In Maturity Model*, BSIMM4 edition, September 2012.
35. T. Mitre Corporation. Common vulnerabilities and exposures.
36. S. J. Murdoch, S. Drimer, R. Anderson, and M. Bond. Chip and PIN is broken. In *Proc. IEEE Symposium on Security and Privacy (SP)*, May 2010.
37. K. Nohl, D. Evans, Starbug, and H. Plötz. Reverse-engineering a cryptographic RFID tag. In *Proceedings of the 17th USENIX Security Symposium*, pages 185–194, July 2008.
38. S. O'Driscoll, A. Poon, and T. Meng. A mm-sized implantable power receiver with adaptive link compensation. In *Proceedings of the International Solid-State Circuits Conference*, ISSCC '09, pages 294–295,295a. IEEE, February 2009.
39. N. Paul, T. Kohno, and D. C. Klonoff. A review of the security of insulin pump infusion systems. *Journal of Diabetes Science and Technology*, 5(6):1557–1562, November 2011.
40. K. Poulsen. Hackers assault epilepsy patients via computer. Wired.com, http://www.wired.com/politics/security/news/2008/03/epilepsy, March 2008.
41. J. Rabaey, M. Mark, D. Chen, C. Sutardja, C. Tang, S. Gowda, M. Wagner, and D. Werthimer. Powering and communicating with mm-size implants. In *Design, Automation & Test in Europe Conference & Exhibition*, DATE '11. IEEE, 2011.
42. J. Radcliffe. Hacking medical devices for fun and insulin: Breaking the human SCADA system. Black Hat Conference presentation slides, August 2011.
43. K. B. Rasmussen, C. Castelluccia, T. S. Heydt-Benjamin, and S. Čapkun. Proximity-based access control for implantable medical devices. In *Proceedings of the 16th ACM Conference on Computer and Communications Security*, pages 410–419, 2009.
44. P. Roberts. Blind attack on wireless insulin pumps could deliver lethal dose. Threatpost (blog post), http://threatpost.com/en_us/blogs/blind-attack-wireless-insulin-pumps-could-deliver-lethal-dose-102711, October 2011.
45. J. Sunshine, S. Egelman, H. Almuhimedi, N. Atri, and L. F. Cranor. Crying wolf: An empirical study of SSL warning effectiveness. In *Proceedings USENIX Security Symposium*, 2009.
46. D. Takahashi. Excuse me while I turn off your insulin pump. VentureBeat, http://venturebeat.com/2011/08/04/excuse-me-while-i-turn-off-your-insulin-pump/, August 2011.
47. U.S. Food and Drug Administration. 510(k) clearances. http://www.fda.gov/medicaldevices/productsandmedicalprocedures/deviceapprovalsandclearances/510kclearances/default.htm, Jun 2009.
48. U.S. Food and Drug Administration. Reminder from FDA: cybersecurity for networked medical devices is a shared responsibility. http://www.fda.gov/MedicalDevices/Safety/AlertsandNotices/ucm189111.htm, Nov. 2009.
49. J. Viega and G. McGraw. *Building Secure Software: How to Avoid Security Problems the Right Way*. Addison-Wesley Professional, 2001.
50. F. Xu, Z. Qin, C. C. Tan, B. Wang, and Q. Li. IMDGuard: Securing implantable medical devices with the external wearable guardian. In *Proceedings of the 30th IEEE International Conference on Computer Communications*, INFOCOM '11, pages 1862–1870, April 2011.

Chapter 8
Attacking and Defending a Diabetes Therapy System

Chunxiao Li, Meng Zhang, Anand Raghunathan, and Niraj K. Jha

Wearable and implantable medical devices are being increasingly deployed to improve diagnosis, monitoring, and therapy for a range of medical conditions.

We demonstrate security attacks that we have implemented in the laboratory on a popular glucose monitoring and insulin delivery system available on the market and also propose defenses against such attacks. Continuous glucose monitoring and insulin delivery systems are becoming increasingly popular among patients with diabetes. These systems utilize wireless communication links, which are frequently exploited as portals to launch security attacks. Our study shows that both passive attacks (eavesdropping on the wireless communication) and active attacks (impersonation and control of the medical devices to alter the intended therapy) can be successfully launched using public-domain information and widely available off-the-shelf hardware. The proposed attacks can compromise both the privacy and safety of patients. We propose three possible defenses against such attacks, which are based on rolling codes, body-coupled communication, and wireless communication monitoring and anomaly detection. The proposed defenses have the potential to greatly mitigate the security risks associated with medical devices.

Introduction

Glucose monitoring and insulin delivery systems are used for the treatment and management of diabetes. In the United States, the Centers for Disease Control and Prevention estimates that 25.8 million people (8.3% of the population) live with

C. Li • M. Zhang • N.K. Jha (✉)
Department of Electrical Engineering, Princeton University
e-mail: chunxiao@princeton.edu; mengz@princeton; jha@princeton.edu

A. Raghunathan
School of Electrical and Computer Engineering, Purdue University
e-mail: raghunathan@purdue.edu

W. Burleson and S. Carrara (eds.), *Security and Privacy for Implantable Medical Devices*, DOI 10.1007/978-1-4614-1674-6_8,

diabetes [1]. Most diabetics use glucose meters, and a rapidly growing number of them are using insulin pumps for therapy. There were around 245,000 insulin pump users in 2005, and the market for insulin pumps is expected to grow at a compound rate of 9% from 2009 to 2016 [5,6].

Continuous glucose monitoring and insulin delivery systems commonly employ wireless communication among their components, such as the glucose monitor, insulin pump, and remote control, connecting them to form a real-time monitoring and response loop. Unfortunately, the wireless channel also serves as a portal to launch security attacks. For example, what if incorrect blood glucose results are sent to the insulin pump wirelessly by malicious attackers? And what if the attackers can control the insulin pump remotely and stop the required insulin injection or inject insulin at a much higher dose than necessary?

These scenarios are not as far-fetched as they may appear. We have analyzed a popular glucose monitoring and insulin delivery system that is currently available on the market. With only the user's manual and some publicly available information, such as the specifications of the radio chip used by the insulin pump, we were able to eavesdrop on the wireless communications using off-the-shelf hardware and a publicly available software radio platform [13]. Since cryptography is not employed, we were able to eavesdrop on the data in a cleartext form. After reverse engineering the communication protocol and packet format, we were able to fully discover the device PIN of the remote control and glucose meter and generate a legitimate data packet, accepted by the insulin pump, containing misleading information, for example, an incorrect reading of the glucose level, control command for stopping/resuming insulin injection, and control command for immediately injecting a dose of insulin into the patient's body. Studies [16] have shown that blood glucose results from miscoded meters may result in significant insulin dose errors. Misconfigured insulin therapy may cause hyperglycemia (high blood glucose) or hypoglycemia (low blood glucose) and endanger the patient's life.

We suggest three possible defenses against security attacks on medical devices. Although they are described in the context of diabetes therapy systems, the proposed defenses are also applicable to many other personal healthcare systems. One solution is to employ cryptography in the communication protocol. However, cryptographic algorithms and protocols used in general-purpose computing platforms are too heavyweight (in terms of processing capability, memory, and power requirements) for many medical devices. Inspired by lightweight cryptographic techniques used in remote-entry systems for automobiles and buildings, we propose the use of rolling-code-based encryption and apply it to the insulin delivery system [13]. We also explore a more novel defense based on the concept of body-coupled communication (BCC), which significantly raises the difficulty for the attacker of eavesdropping on the communication channels used within various components of a personal healthcare system [13]. We experimentally demonstrate the efficacy of BCC compared to a conventional wireless channel. Our third solution is a general framework for securing medical devices based on wireless channel monitoring and anomaly detection. We discuss a medical security monitor (MedMon) that snoops on all the radio-frequency wireless communications to/from medical devices and uses multilayered anomaly detection to identify potentially malicious transactions [19].

Background and Related Work

In this section, we present some background material and related research.

A glucose monitoring and insulin delivery system may consist of several components:

- Glucose meter: there are two types of glucose meter available on the market. The first is the traditional palm-sized meter that uses a test strip and a drop of blood to determine the glucose level, which is then displayed on the meter. Some meters have the ability to transmit the glucose data to a computer for logging or to an insulin pump as a reference for insulin injection. The other type is a blood glucose monitor that samples blood glucose levels on a continual basis, typically every few minutes. The monitor includes a disposable glucose sensor placed under the skin to measure the glucose level and a transmitter attached to the sensor to transmit data to a computer or insulin pump.
- Insulin pen: the manual insulin syringe/pen is a medical device that can inject an accurate insulin dose into the human body. It is currently used by most insulin-treated patients.
- Insulin pump: the insulin pump is a medical device that is used for autonomous administration of insulin through subcutaneous infusion. The pump includes a controlling and processing module, powered by batteries, to program the time, dose, and rate of insulin injection. A disposable insulin reservoir and an infusion set are also included in the pump. The pump delivers insulin in two doses: bolus and basal. A bolus dose is pumped quickly through a normal injection to account for the food eaten or to correct a high blood glucose level. For a bolus dose, the injection time, rate, and dose can be adjusted based on the patient's needs, such as the number of meals or consumption of highly glycemic foods. A basal dose is slowly and continuously injected at an adjustable rate between meals and at night. Its injection time, rate, and dose can also be programmed based on the patient's needs, such as a rate reduction at night for infants and a rate increase for teenagers due to the presence of growth hormone. In some "smart" insulin pumps, bolus calculators are embedded in the pump to help users calculate the dose for the next insulin bolus based on the amount of carbohydrates consumed, which is entered by the user manually.

  Four different programming and communication interfaces are implemented on current insulin pumps: (1) buttons on the pump itself, (2) wireless connection to a remote control, (3) wireless connection to a computer, used to upload data or manage the programming, and (4) wireless connection to a blood glucose monitor.
- Remote control: a remote control is a device that controls and programs the insulin pump. A full-featured remote control can do all the programming required by the insulin pump, whereas a simple remote control might only allow the user to deliver a discrete bolus dose or stop/resume insulin delivery.

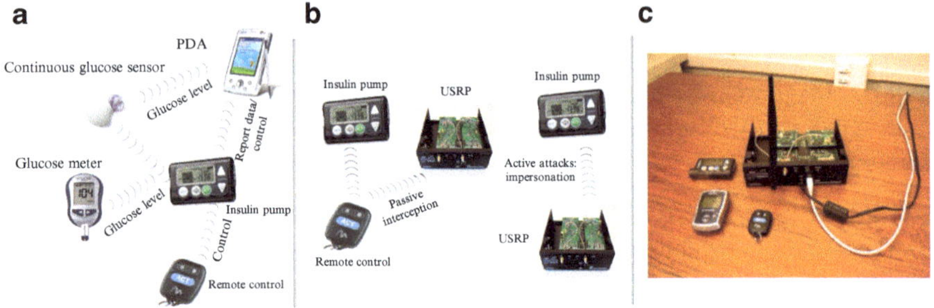

Fig. 8.1 (**a**) Insulin delivery system, (**b**) security attacks, and (**c**) experimental setup used in the attacks

- Personal health hub: smartphones or computers may be used to log data from the continuous blood glucose monitor, blood glucose meter, and insulin pump, organize and visualize the data, and report them to the patient and doctor for improved therapy management.

Diabetics are increasingly migrating from the traditional glucose meter and manual insulin injection systems to continuous glucose monitoring and automatic insulin delivery systems since they offer greater convenience and better control over blood glucose levels. In the traditional system, patients read data from the glucose meter and inject insulin using the insulin syringe/pen. However, convenience and better control over blood glucose levels are increasingly driving the adoption of continuous glucose monitoring and insulin delivery systems.

In a recent study, patients who wore insulin pumps for continuous insulin injection reported a better quality of life than when using other devices [2]. In such systems, as shown in Fig. 8.1a, there exist several wireless links to automate the process: the link from the meter/monitor to the pump to transmit glucose levels and the link from the remote control or computer to the pump to transmit control commands. These wireless links are security-critical to the whole insulin delivery system—they impact confidentiality, integrity, and availability. However, the wireless links in currently available glucose monitoring and insulin delivery systems may be insecure. We specifically show how to successfully intercept and attack the wireless links using off-the-shelf hardware and software and show how these attacks may then be used to undermine the correct operation of the insulin delivery system and endanger the patient's life.

Several previous research efforts have reported the adverse effects of accidental software and hardware failures [12] as well as human errors [16] in medical devices. However, it is only recently that malicious attacks against these devices have been considered and demonstrated. Our work is the first demonstration of a malicious attack on a real glucose monitoring and insulin delivery system. Since we first published our attacks in June 2011 [13], other researchers have also shown the feasibility of attacks on insulin pumps [4, 15].

The previous effort closest to our research [11] demonstrated attacks on pacemakers and implantable cardiac defibrillators and proposed zero-power defenses.

Although similar in overall objectives, our work differs significantly in the attack methodology and proposed defenses. As the authors stated in [11], they did not perform packet analysis or reassembly, "only simple waveform manipulation and repetition." We, however, fully reverse engineered the radio protocol of the insulin delivery system so that adversaries could reassemble the packets and emulate the full functions of a remote control: wake up the insulin pump, stop/resume the insulin injection, or immediately inject a bolus dose of insulin into the human body. The defenses that we propose are all different from those presented in [11].

Defense solutions proposed for pacemakers and implantable cardiac defibrillators include IMDGuardian [17] and the "shield" [10]. All of our defenses differ from the aforementioned proposals. Our proposal for wireless monitoring and anomaly detection also relies on an external device. However, our solution is applicable to communication links between medical devices (e.g., glucose monitor and insulin pump) as well as links between medical devices and external programmers. In contrast, previous proposals only target the links between medical devices and external programmers. Moreover, we do not require the complex design of a full-duplex radio or even changes to external programmers. Thus, we believe that our solutions either complement or are attractive alternatives to previous proposals.

Passive and Active Attacks

We next discuss successful passive and active attacks on a commercially available insulin delivery system. Our experimental setup includes a glucose meter, an insulin pump, a remote control, and a Universal Software Radio Peripheral (USRP) [7]. We choose not to fully disclose the product information (brand, type, and model number) here since the system that we analyze is currently in use by patients.

USRP is an off-the-shelf software radio board that currently costs around $700. With free software (GNU radio [3]) and appropriate daughter boards, the USRP can intercept radio communications within a frequency band and generate wireless signals with different configurations of data, frequency, modulation, and power.

As shown in Fig. 8.1b, we focused on the wireless link from the remote control to the insulin pump and intercepted the communication. We then fully reverse engineered the communication protocol and were able to successfully launch active attacks that remotely controlled the insulin pump. We show the experimental setup in Fig. 8.1c.

Frequency

The operating frequency of the wireless link needs to be determined first. The frequency of any wireless device is publicly available online and easily obtained through its Federal Communications Commission (FCC) ID. In our example system,

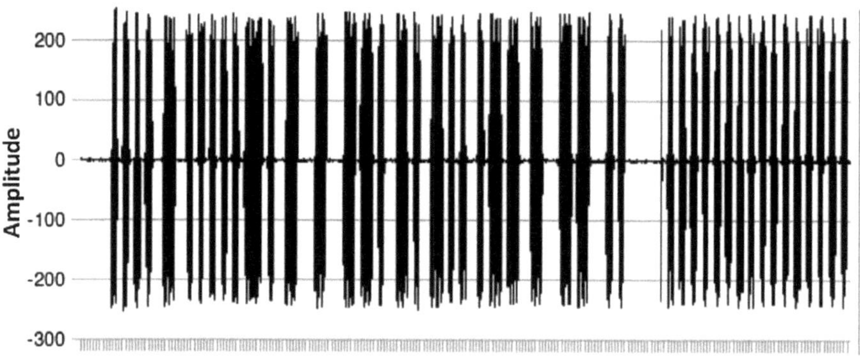

Fig. 8.2 Signal intercepted by USRP

the communication between the remote control and insulin pump uses 915 MHz frequency. A 915 MHz daughter board and antenna are attached to the USRP board to receive and generate a signal in the 915 MHz frequency band.

Modulation Type

We intercepted the wireless signal around 915 MHz and down-converted it to near the baseband, as shown in Fig. 8.2. After analysis, we found that on–off keying was used in the communication. This modulation scheme uses the presence of a carrier wave to indicate a binary 1 and its absence to indicate a binary 0.

Packet Format

For both the glucose meter and remote control, in order to make the insulin pump receive the data or control command, a code of six hexadecimal digits needs to be entered into the insulin pump manually by users. The digits are printed on the back of a glucose meter or remote control as a personal identification number (PIN). We ascertained that not entering the PIN or entering the wrong PIN caused a failed communication. However, as explained below, the PIN is transmitted in plaintext and can be captured by simply eavesdropping on the communication between the devices.

We intercepted the data packets from the remote control (generated by different buttons) to the glucose meter. After the synchronizing sequence of 0s and 1s, there were 80 information bits. We deciphered these bits after a thorough analysis: (1) the first 4 bits represent the device type because they are different when different types of devices are used (glucose meters or remote controls), (2) the next 36 bits constitute the device PIN because they are different for each device, and (3) the last

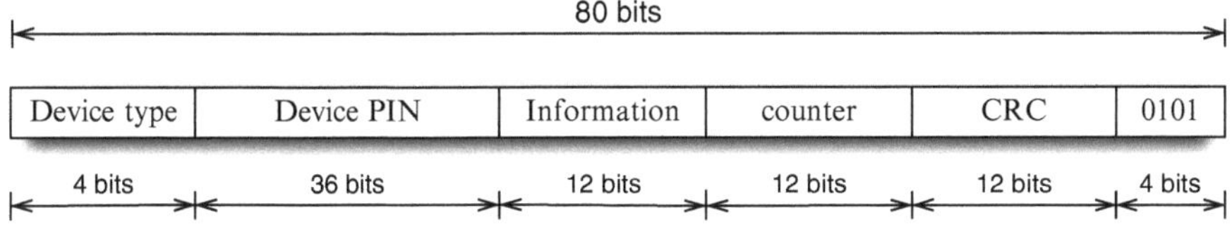

Fig. 8.3 Format of communication packet in insulin delivery system

40 bits can be split into four parts: the first 12 bits are payload bits indicating which button was pressed or what glucose level reading was transmitted; the next 12 bits are counters and repeat after 256 counts; the next 12 bits seem random but actually perform a cyclic redundancy check (CRC); the last 4 bits are always 0101.

After more testing and analysis, we were finally able to parse the communication packet, in the format shown in Fig. 8.3.

Counter and CRC

After identifying the 12-bit counter, we found the pattern that it repeats after 256 counts—which means it is actually an 8-bit counter. We treated it like a two-digit hexadecimal counter that counts from 00 to FF. This indicates that a sequence of 6 bits may represent a hexadecimal digit—an increasing count of two hexadecimal digits repeats after 256 counts. We then constructed a correspondence table between the bits in the communication packet and the corresponding hexadecimal digits. We found that the device PIN was actually sent in cleartext without any encryption—every PIN digit was represented by 6 bits based on this correspondence table and the 36 PIN bits represented six hexadecimal digits printed on the back of the medical device. For security reasons, we choose not to disclose the mapping between the information bits and hexadecimal digits.

The 12 bits next to the counter are for CRC. CRC computation is based on polynomial division. In practice, the CRC algorithm divides a binary string by the *generator polynomial* string, where subtraction is replaced by exclusive-OR operations.

The sender (remote control in this case) calculates a short, fixed-length binary sequence (12 bits in this case) for each block of data and sends them together as a packet. When a packet is received, the device repeats the calculation using the same CRC algorithm. If the calculated CRC does not match the one received, the data may contain a transmission error and the packet is dropped. Several parameters are involved in the CRC calculation:

- CRC order: this is the order of the CRC polynomial.
- CRC polynomial: this is the polynomial used in the division of the binary strings. It is often represented by a hexadecimal string counted without the leading 1 bit. For example, a common polynomial for 8-bit CRC is 0×07, which means the polynomial is $x^8 + x^2 + x + 1$.

Table 8.1 CRC parameters for remote control and glucose meter

Parameters	Remote control	Glucose meter
CRC order	8	8
CRC polynomial	*x*	*x*
Initial value	0	0
Final XOR value	*x*	*x*
Reverse data bytes	N	N
Reverse CRC result	N	N

- Initial value: this is the value to exclusive-OR with the binary string before division.
- Final XOR value: this is the value to exclusive-OR with the final results of division.
- Reverse data bytes: these indicate whether the data bytes are reversed before division.
- Reverse CRC result: this indicates whether the result of CRC is reversed before matching.

After many trials, we were able to find the CRC parameters used in the insulin delivery system considered here. Note that these parameters are needed if we want to generate a legitimate packet with our own information bits that is acceptable to the insulin pump because packets without the correct CRC will be dropped. In Table 8.1, we show the parameters of the CRC for both the remote control and glucose meter (they use similar CRC parameters). For security reasons, some of the parameter values are replaced with "*x*."

Replay

The system employs a simple security mechanism to defend against replay attacks: a packet is not accepted if its counter has exactly the same value as the last packet. However, we found that as long as the counter has a different value from the last one, the packet is accepted. Therefore, we were able to intercept two packets and transmit them in an alternating fashion. Replaying the information can be done for simple attacks, such as reporting an outdated glucose level to the insulin pump.

Generation of Arbitrary Packets

Having determined the format of the packet and the parameters of the CRC, it is now possible to generate a legitimate packet that will be accepted by the insulin pump. We performed tests on the real system by entering a new random device PIN into the pump and generating a new control packet using this PIN. We were able to fully control the insulin pump using the USRP as a remote control.

Attack Scenarios

Next, we analyze possible practical attack scenarios based on the attacks presented in the previous section. The attack scenarios are categorized into two groups, which are discussed in the next two subsections.

Attacks Without Knowledge of the Device PIN

If the attacker does not know the device PIN of the remote control or glucose monitor, some of the possible attacks are as follows:

- **Privacy attacks**. Eavesdropping on any wireless link in the insulin delivery system considered here would expose (1) the existence of the therapy and glucose level, and thus the medical condition of the patient, (2) the device type, and (3) the device PIN, which will give the attacker an open door to launch all the attacks discussed in the next group.
- **Integrity attacks**. Even without knowledge of the device PIN, using the alternating transmission of two consecutive packets, the attacker can still control the insulin pump or report an incorrect (past) glucose reading to the insulin pump. More details are given in what follows.
- **Availability attacks**. Attackers can simply jam the communication channel between the medical devices, causing incorrect operation. However, these attacks can be easily detected by the patient: either the remote control does not work or the data transmission fails.

Attacks with Knowledge of the Device PIN

If the attacker knows the device PIN of the remote control (glucose meter) of the insulin pump, either by reading the printed device PIN from the medical device or using the eavesdropping attacks discussed earlier, other attacks that can be launched are as follows: (1) one could stop insulin injection into the human body, which will cause a high glucose level, (2) one could resume insulin injection into the human body if it is currently stopped, or (3) one could inject a bolus dose into the human body, which may lead to hypoglycemia and endanger the patient's life.

We have not verified that the format of the communication protocol between the continuous glucose monitor and the insulin pump is the same as that between the remote control and pump discussed earlier. However, we believe that one could easily attack this wireless link using the same methodology. If the attacker knows the device PIN of the continuous glucose monitor, he can report a false reading to the pump and mislead the patient into injecting more or less insulin than needed. This attack is less feasible if a traditional glucose meter with a display is used because the user can always verify whether the two readings are the same. However, since the continuous glucose monitor is attached to the human skin and no display is available, this attack can be more easily launched.

Besides intercepting the communication on the wireless link first, attackers also have other means for obtaining the device PIN, such as peeking at the printed PIN or through insider information from the device manufacturer or supply chain.

Attack Experiments

First, we set up and evaluated the passive attack scenario: while the remote control was communicating with the insulin pump, we eavesdropped on the signal and measured the signal strength (amplitude in Fig. 8.2) using the USRP eavesdropping device at different distances from the remote control. We concluded that within 7–8 m, the signal strength was well above the noise level and it was easy to eavesdrop on the signals and extract the device type, device PIN, and the control command sent to the insulin pump. Since the maximum attacking distance depends on the antenna and the sensitivity of the receiver, we believe that a better antenna and receiver chip could extend this distance further.

Second, we set up the active attack scenario: we used the USRP to control the insulin pump from a distance. We used the device PIN extracted from the last step to generate some unauthenticated control commands. We verified that using the maximum allowed the power level of the USRP daughter board, which is 200 mW (23 dB), the insulin pump accepted commands to control and stop/resume insulin injection that were sent from a distance of greater than 20 m. We believe that, with a better antenna and larger output power, even larger active attack distances could be achieved.

In conclusion, using an off-the-shelf device, such as the USRP, passive and active attacks on the insulin delivery system considered here are possible. For example, in a hospital, an attacker can eavesdrop and extract the device PIN of the remote control from outside a patient's room at a distance of 7–8 m and secretly control insulin injection even from 20 m away.

Defending Against Security Attacks

In this section, we discuss three possible defenses against attacks on medical devices and describe them in the context of the diabetes therapy system.

One simple and obvious solution is to use cryptography, yet it is frequently not used, in part due to the impact on battery life. A very similar scenario for the insulin delivery system considered here is automobile keyless entry. Both have the following characteristics: one-way communication, very low data rate, and high

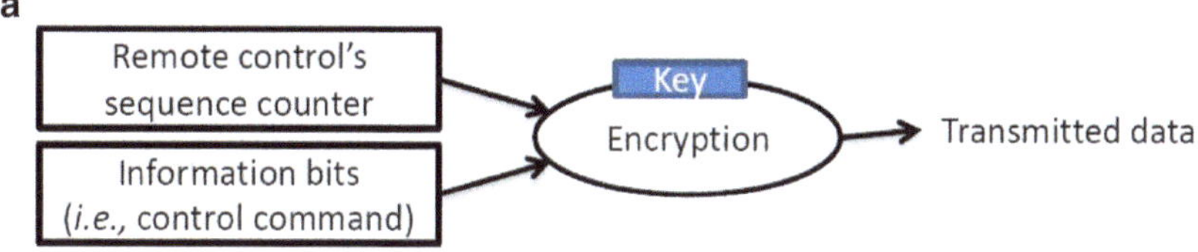

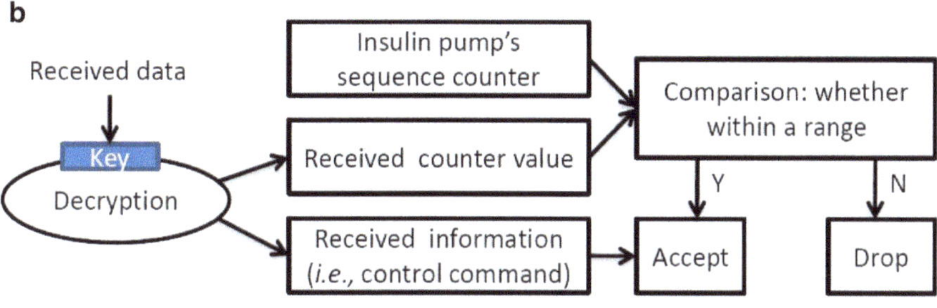

Fig. 8.4 Proposed rolling code encoder/decoder in insulin delivery system

security requirements. We refer to the current security protocols in automobile keyless entry systems and propose their application to the diabetes therapy system.

Another more general solution is to use BCC in the system to avoid attacks from the lowermost physical layer. We introduce the principles of BCC and, for the first time, show experimental results related to the security of BCC and its implications on body-area medical device networks.

A third solution is a medical security monitor (MedMon) that snoops on all the radio-frequency wireless communications to/from medical devices and uses multilayered anomaly detection to identify potentially malicious transactions.

Cryptographic Approach

Instead of sending a fixed device PIN every time, rolling codes are widely used in automobile keyless entry systems [8]. Based on this technique, we propose a rolling code encoder embedded in the remote control and a rolling code decoder in the insulin pump, as shown in Fig. 8.4.

The remote control and insulin pump share an encryption key. The key in the remote control is used to encrypt a number in the sequence counter. The number is increased by 1 for every communication packet. In the insulin pump, the encrypted data are decrypted using the shared key and the decrypted sequence number is compared to the receiver's counter. If the difference is within a certain range (the remote control may have had several failed communications previously), the insulin pump believes that the received control code is valid, synchronizes the sequence counter, and performs the task.

With the rolling code technique, it becomes impossible for attackers to simply extract the device PIN or to launch replay attacks because the transmitted data are encrypted and the rolling code changes every time. The security of the rolling code system depends on the encryption/decryption algorithm and the encryption keys. Previous research [14] has shown successful attacks on one popular encryption block cypher—KeeLoq, used in rolling code systems. These are mainly brute-force attacks, implemented on a cost-optimized parallel code breaker. The secret key of the KeeLoq algorithm is revealed in less than 0.5 s if a 32-bit seed is used and in less than 6 h in the case of a 48-bit seed. The authors argued that a 60-bit seed should be used, for which their code breaker needs about 1,011 days for key recovery in the worst case.

Body-Coupled Communication

Another promising technology that can be used is BCC. We first introduce the BCC technology and then present some BCC-based experimental results to show how the insulin delivery system considered here can be protected.

Introduction to BCC

BCC [9] is a technology that uses the human body as the transmission medium to enable wireless communication, in contrast to the conventional over-the-air communication. One claimed advantage of BCC [9] is that the communication range is limited to the close proximity of the human body, which prevents interference between BCC-based body area networks. Another key advantage is that BCC may consume less power because the data are only sent around the body rather than through free space [18].

In the insulin delivery system considered here, all devices are attached to the body: the continuous glucose meter and the insulin pump need to be directly attached for monitoring and injection; the remote control buttons also need to be pressed and thus are connected to the skin while communicating. If BCC is limited to the close proximity of the human body, not only would the attacks described earlier be useless, but some other attacks could also be eliminated, such as the unauthorized or accidental use of the remote control, as long as the attacker is not very close to the patient or touching the patient's skin.

Previous work provided various measurements [9] for BCC, such as propagation loss as a function of frequency, transceiver position, and electrode size. We focus more on the security of BCC and design experiments to show how BCC can defend against the passive and active attacks described earlier.

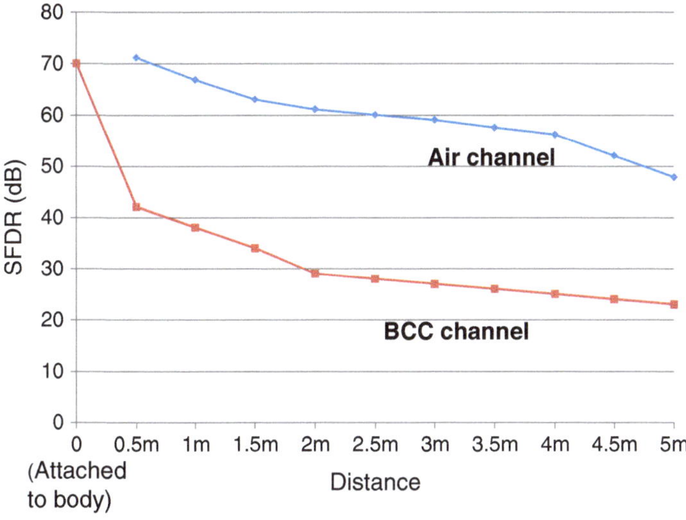

Fig. 8.5 SFDR as a function of distance using air and BCC channels in the case of passive attacks

Experiments

The equipment used in the experiments includes a function generator, a middle-wave/short-wave active loop antenna, electrodes, and USRP.

The first group of experiments is set up to discover which frequency band for BCC causes the least propagation loss. We use the USRP as a receiver and the function generator as a transmitter that transmits a mono-frequency signal. Both are directly connected to the human body via electrodes. The USRP performs a fast Fourier transform on the received signal and the spur-free dynamic range (SFDR) is measured. SFDR is the strength ratio of the fundamental signal to the strongest spurious signal in the output and is a measure of the signal strength relative to the noise level. We decided to use the frequency of 5 MHz, which has a maximum SFDR of 84 dB (with a function generator output peak-to-peak amplitude of 200 mV), as the BCC transmission frequency in the following experiments.

The second group of experiments is set up to show how BCC can defend against passive eavesdropping attacks. We use the function generator to generate a 5 MHz signal, attached to the human body. The USRP mimics the eavesdropping attacker and picks up the signal from some distance. To receive better signals, we use an active-loop antenna in the corresponding frequency band. The results are shown in Fig. 8.5. The original insulin delivery system is also experimentally evaluated for comparison. We adjust the output power of the function generator to enable a fair comparison between BCC and the original air channel: the SFDR of the BCC is the same as that of the remote control signal at a distance of 0.5 m (a typical distance during the normal usage of an insulin delivery system).

The third group of experiments is set up to show how the BCC can defend against active attacks. We use a function generator equipped with an antenna to

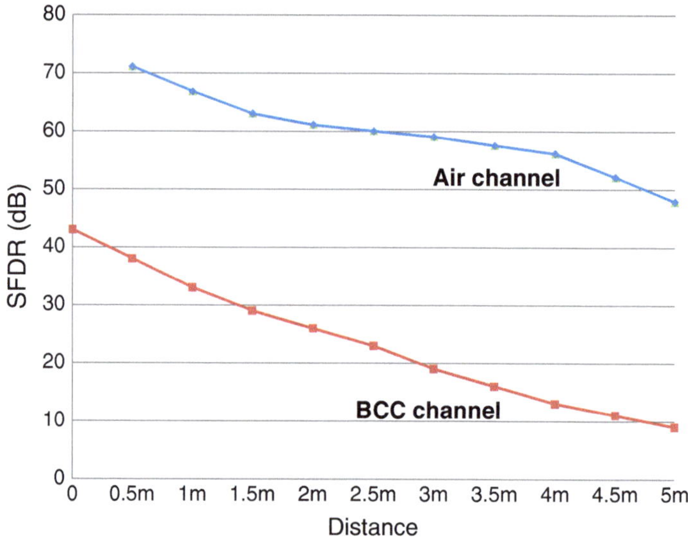

Fig. 8.6 SFDR as a function of distance using air and BCC channels in the case of active attacks

broadcast the signal, and then use the USRP, which is attached to the human body via electrodes, to pick up the signal. The function generator mimics the active attacker trying to control the medical device and the device attached to the body receives the signals. The results are shown in Fig. 8.6. The original insulin delivery system is also evaluated for comparison.

From the experiments we can conclude that BCC does help mitigate passive and active attacks: for passive eavesdropping attacks, at the same distance, the SFDR of the signal is around 30 dB less than in the case of conventional communication, making the signal more difficult to eavesdrop on; for active attacks, the strength of the received signal from the human body is also much less (30–40 dB) than in the case of conventional communication, making it more difficult to control the insulin pump from some distance away.

However, note that the SFDR of the received signal also depends on the antenna and the output power of the transmitter. Therefore, even though the foregoing experiments show that BCC can help mitigate the security problem, experiments need to be performed for each device in the different attack scenarios in order to confirm the security enhancement.

MedMon: Securing Medical Devices Through Wireless Monitoring and Anomaly Detection

MedMon is a wearable external device that defends medical devices against malicious attacks [19]. At a high level, MedMon is similar to a network firewall

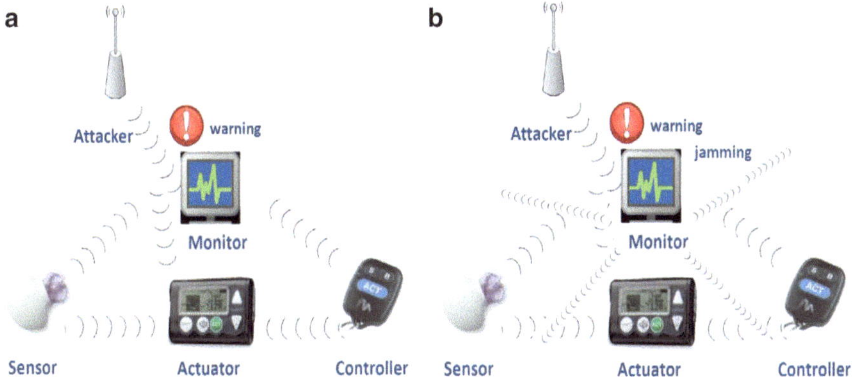

Fig. 8.7 Upon identifying an attack, MedMon (**a**) just provides a warning in the passive mode, (**b**) provides a warning and jams the communication in the active mode

in that it analyzes all communication traffic to/from the secured device, searches for anomalies in the communication traffic, and blocks communication that it deems malicious. However, unlike traditional network firewalls, MedMon operates at the physical and application layers due to the characteristics of medical devices and their communications.

The operation of MedMon is illustrated in Fig. 8.7. When anomalies are identified, indicating a possible attack, the monitor can respond passively or actively, depending on its configuration for this type of anomaly or attack. The monitor is set to the passive (active) mode for a particular anomaly if the potential damage is low (high). In the passive mode, it provides a warning to the patient through an alarm or vibration, without interfering with ongoing communication. In the active mode, in addition to alerting the patient, it interferes with the transmission by sending jamming signals, so that the suspicious transmission is blocked before it can complete and succeed in altering the state of the devices. To accommodate different devices and patient needs, the monitor needs to be trained and configured first in order to learn the characteristics of normal behavior.

Layered Anomaly Detection

MedMon uses a layered approach to anomaly detection, wherein information from the physical and application layers is used to detect potentially malicious communication. The layers of anomaly detection are in Fig. 8.8. The outer layers, i.e., the physical indicators, are examined first. If the transmitted signal passes the anomaly detection in the outer layers, the monitor searches for data or command anomalies in the underlying content. If no anomaly is found, the communication is deemed safe and allowed to proceed.

We next discuss the anomaly detection in further detail.

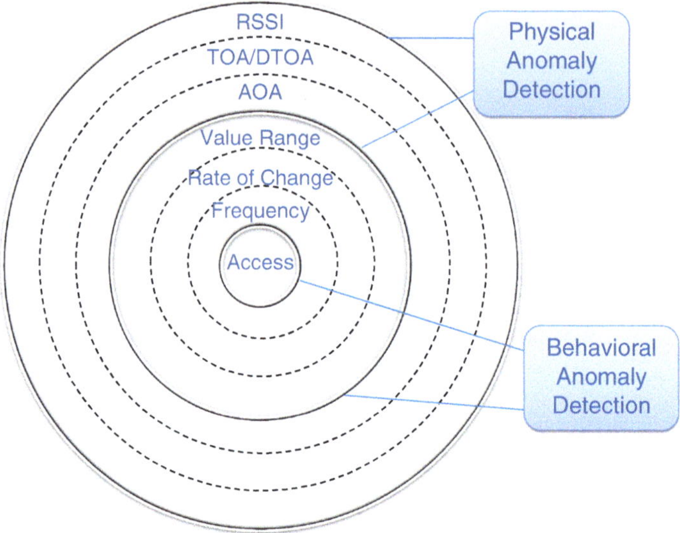

Fig. 8.8 Layers of anomaly detection in MedMon

Physical Anomalies

MedMon starts its examination by observing the physical characteristics of the transmitted signal. Such characteristics may include the received signal strength indicator (RSSI), time of arrival (TOA), differential time of arrival (DTOA), and angle of arrival (AOA). In radiolocation, RSSI, TOA, and DTOA are used to estimate the distance of a transmitter from the receiver, and AOA is used to determine the transmitter's direction in relation to the receiver. Knowing these characteristics of the transmitter allows the monitor to verify its legitimacy with high confidence.

- **RSSI**: if the distance between the monitor and each transmitting device is known and expected to remain relatively constant, the signal strength from the device can be expected to fall within a specific range. An anomaly is detected if the signal allegedly sent by the device has unusually high or low strength.
- **TOA**: if a transmission is scheduled to occur at specific points in time, the occurrence of the transmission at a nonscheduled time reveals an anomaly.
- **DTOA**: if a transmission is scheduled to occur periodically at certain time intervals, early arrival of the transmission signal is recognized as an anomaly.
- **AOA**: assuming the monitor is carried at a fixed location on the patient, e.g., attached to the right side of the patient's belt, a transmitting device, e.g., a sensor on the patient's back, will have a fixed angle relative to MedMon. In such cases, AOA could be used to examine whether the signal is arriving from the correct direction. For example, the monitor will report an anomaly if it receives sensor signals from the front, when it expects them to come from the back.

Behavioral Anomalies

An examination of physical indicators cannot guarantee that all attacks will be caught. For example, attack signals might have the physical characteristics that satisfy all requirements by chance or through sophisticated design. However, although an attack signal may be physically indistinguishable from a normal signal, the underlying information (commands or data) can typically be distinguished due to its intention to cause harm to the patient, e.g., a malicious command that orders repeated or large-dose drug injections or forged data that feign sudden changes in vital signs to induce unnecessary drug delivery.

We define anomalies in the underlying information to be behavioral anomalies. The monitor keeps a record of the historical data and commands. When new commands/data arrive, it compares them to the historical record to decide whether the new commands/data constitute a behavioral anomaly.

When a command anomaly is detected, such as for repeated drug injections, the monitor prevents the new command from being executed by jamming the command signal in order to protect patient health and safety. If the command is authorized by the patient, the patient can simply revise the command or change the anomaly definition in the monitor's configuration.

When a data anomaly is detected, such as a sudden change in the patient's vital signs, the monitor raises a warning. Abnormal data may be generated by an attacker or may actually represent deteriorating patient condition. In either case, the monitor's warning alerts the patient to an attack or a health condition that he/she should be concerned about.

Security Policies

Anomalies can be defined within security policies. Security policies define what the monitor's response should be to each detected anomaly. Each transmitting device has its own set of security policies. The monitor is guided by the security policies of the transmitting device when snooping on its transmission.

During the training period, the patient carries the monitor, with the medical devices operating normally. After collecting a sufficient number of values for RSSI, TOA, DTOA, and AOA for each transmitting device, the monitor determines if each parameter has values that fall in a certain range and, if so, decides the thresholds for the parameter. If a parameter does not have a range of normal values, it is not included in the device's security policies.

Summary

In this chapter, we discussed security and privacy issues related to a current diabetes therapy system. We showed that through reverse engineering of the radio protocols, both passive and active attacks can be launched on a commercial insulin delivery system using off-the-shelf hardware and software. We then analyzed the various attack scenarios and proposed three types of defense against them. We believe that the proposed attack methodology and defenses are applicable to several wearable and implantable medical devices. Although promising advances have been made in the field, medical device security remains a critical challenge that demands the immediate attention of the research community.

Acknowledgements This work was supported by the National Science Foundation in part under Grant NSF CNS-0914787 and in part under CNS-1219570.

References

1. 2007 national diabetes fact sheet, http://www.cdc.gov/diabetes/pubs/pdf/ndfs_2011.pdf.
2. Experiences with insulin pump in 52 patients, http://professional.diabetes.org/abstracts_display.aspx?typ=1&cid=70361.
3. GNU radio, http://www.gnu.org/software/gnuradio/.
4. Hacker shows off lethal attack by controlling wireless medical device, http://go.bloomberg.com/tech-blog/2012-02-29-hacker-shows-off-lethal-attack-by-controlling-wireless-medical-device/.
5. Insulin pumps - global pipeline analysis, opportunity assessment and market forecasts to 2016, http://www.globaldata.com.
6. US healthcare equipment and supplies – diabetes, http://www.research.hsbc.com.
7. USRP, http://www.ettus.com/.
8. A. I. Alrabady and S. M. Mahmud. Analysis of attacks against the security of keyless-entry systems for vehicles and suggestions for improved designs. *IEEE Trans. Vehicular Technology*, 54:41–50, Jan. 2005.
9. H. Baldus, S. Corroy, A. Fazzi, K. Klabunde, and T. Schenk. Human-centric connectivity enabled by body-coupled communications. *IEEE Communications Magazine*, 47:172–178, June 2009.
10. S. Gollakota, H. Hassanieh, B. Ransford, D. Katabi, and K. Fu. They can hear your heartbeats: Non-invasive security for implantable medical devices. In *Proc. ACM Conf. Special Interest Group on Data Communication*, Aug. 2011.
11. D. Halperin, T. S. Heydt-Benjamin, B. Ransford, S. S. Clark, B. Defend, W. Morgan, K. Fu, T. Kohno, and W. H. Maisel. Pacemakers and implantable cardiac defibrillators: Software radio attacks and zero-power defenses. In *Proc. IEEE Symp. Security and Privacy*, pages 129–142, May 2008.
12. N. G. Leveson and C. S. Turner. An investigation of the Therac-25 accidents. *Computer*, 26: 18–41, July 1993.
13. C. Li, A. Raghunathan, and N. K. Jha. Hijacking an insulin pump: Security attacks and defenses for a diabetes therapy system. In *Proc. IEEE Int. Conf. on e-Health Networking Applications and Services*, pages 150–156, June 2011.
14. M. Novotny and T. Kasper. Cryptanalysis of KeeLoq with COPACOBANA. In *Proc. Wkshp. Special Purpose Hardware for Attacking Cryptographic Systems*, pages 159–164, Sept. 2009.
15. J. Radcliffe. Hacking medical devices for fun and insulin: Breaking the human SCADA System. In *Proc. Black Hat Technical Security Conference*, July-Aug. 2011.
16. C. H. Raine, L. E. Schrock, S. V. Edelman, S. R. Mudaliar, W. Zhong, L. J. Proud, and J. L. Parkes. Significant insulin dose errors may occur if blood glucose results are obtained from miscoded meters. *J. Diabetes Science and Technology*, 1(2):205–210, Mar. 2007.

17. F. Xu, Z. Qin, C. C. Tan, B. Wang, and Q. Li. IMDGuard: Securing implantable medical devices with the external wearable guardian. In *Proc. IEEE Int. Conf. Computer Communications*, pages 1862–1870, Apr. 2011.
18. H.-J. Yoo, S.-J. Song, N. Cho, and H.-J. Kim. Low energy on-body communication for BSN. In *Proc. Int. Wkshp. Wearable and Implantable Body Sensor Networks*, pages 15–20, Mar. 2007.
19. M. Zhang, A. Raghunathan, and N. K. Jha. MedMon: Securing medical devices through wireless monitoring and anomaly detection. *IEEE Trans. on Biomedical Circuits and Systems*, accepted for publication.

Chapter 9
Conclusions and A Vision of the Future

Sandro Carrara and Wayne Burleson

In summary, this short book has provided a brief introduction to the new research area of security and privacy in the field of implantable medical devices (IMDs) by presenting two sides of the problem, namely, IMDs and embedded security. The book has four chapters written by international leaders in the field of implantable medical devices [1]. These chapters introduce the latest advances and research problems in the area of IMDs. The first chapter is from an industry leader in the field of implantable devices for continuous glucose monitoring. Their subcutaneous system for glucose sampling is described in the chapter and the whole monitoring system is presented, including a palm device that wirelessly connects the sensors. This provides the first clear example in the book of a system that is already on the market and that presents a potential vulnerability for malicious attacks (the wireless connection between the handheld reader of the physician and the sensory device wore by the patient). The next two chapters are from scientists in two leading academic institutions (one in the United States and the other in Europe). These chapters present more advanced research results from the scientific literature concerning the monitoring of several metabolites (molecules related to metabolic states) for different applications in both unhealthy and healthy patients. These chapters show two different systems, recently published in the literature, that contain more than one sensor and that, therefore, could monitor several metabolites simultaneously. In both cases, the sensory device is a subcutaneous implant that is remotely connected with a device located externally with respect to the body. Therefore, a potential eavesdropping or impersonation vulnerability arises again,

S. Carrara (✉)
École polytechnique fédérale de Lausanne, Lausanne, Switzerland
e-mail: Sandro.carrara@epfl.ch

W. Burleson
Department of Electrical and Computer Engineering, University of Massachusetts,
309C Knowles Engineering Building, Amherst 01003, USA
e-mail: Burleson@ecs.umass.edu

W. Burleson and S. Carrara (eds.), *Security and Privacy for Implantable Medical Devices*,
DOI 10.1007/978-1-4614-1674-6_9,

although reduced due to the short-range communication. The removability of the external device raises authentication and privacy concerns. The last chapter dedicated to implantable medical devices focuses on a new approach that is currently under development in regenerative medicine: the possibility of inserting in the body a bioreactor that might regenerate damaged tissue directly in the body region of interest. Of course, the future development of this extremely fascinating approach to regenerating human organs foresees the introduction of sensors and actuators that allow a deeper and closer control of bioreactors. Again, remote sensing and control of a bioreactor requires a reliable and secure channel for data communication and operation commands. Hopefully these four examples provide a background on the possibilities of IMDs, as well as the potential vulnerabilities and motivations for a malicious attack.

From the security side, the book has also presented two chapters on recent attacks and potential defensive solutions (often called counter-measures). Chapter 7 has showed potential attacks against a Diabetes Therapy System and how to develop a robust defending device to protect it. The final chapter, Chap. 8 discusses Insulin System, Pacemaker, and Sub-cutaneous Biosensor as three examples of IMDs with significant security and privacy requirements. The chapter looks at each and proposes challenges, solutions, and open problems. It also presents more general issues and approaches to systematic design of secure Implantable Medical Devices.

A Vision of the Future

As we have seen in this book, IMDs present exciting opportunities for the future by opening up possibilities that were just science fiction a few years ago. In the future, the full monitoring of human metabolism in a minimally invasive and remote manner will be possible thanks to robust, reliable, and low-cost systems. The availability of these systems will allow an unprecedented capability for patient diagnostics and monitoring. It will also open new approaches to personalized medicine, which had been envisioned in the past [2] but could not be implemented due to a lack of cost-effective sensing technology. The field is now growing rapidly, and new technologies [3] have overcome many of the hurdles for implantable devices, including sensitivity, differentiation, energy issues, biocompatibility, and, to some extent, security and privacy. But challenges in all of these areas remain.

Unlike many objects on the Internet of Things, new implantable devices for personalized medicine, which might include both sensors and actuators, require security due to their applications to human health and safety. Moreover, the sensitivity of the data collected on the health status of each individual case requires special care in terms of data privacy and protection. Therefore, we have outlined some of the design challenges and solutions in the book's second section, which is focused on systems for security and privacy. Much work remains to be done and, thus the future presents a charge to research communities to conduct further investigations and pursue more developments, both in terms of new technologies and an awareness of existing and emerging technologies from both sides. To show this future trend, what follows are recommendations on policy and governance issues surrounding future IMDs.

The present state of the art in implantable technology has little to offer in terms of data security and privacy. Sensing technology seems to be ready for the next step to acquire, integrate, and transmit biological data on the status not only of patients but also people interested in fitness (e.g., athletes) as well. However, current policy on this possible development is still in the early stages regarding legislation on privacy and security. More often, the implantable devices on the market do not foresee any system on board that could address security and privacy needs. On the other hand, society is aware of the security and privacy issues related in other areas of everyday life. Therefore, there is also increasing awareness in the field of medical data and, with increasing attention from the scientific community, in the field of fully IMDs.

From this perspective, it is clear that over the next 3 to 5 years researchers and technologists need to consider more extensively the privacy and security issues related to IMDs. The reasons for this are manifold: we would like to see on the market many distributed medical and diagnostic devices (portable, wearable, implantable, etc.), we would like to have robust technologies that allow for precision in the monitoring and control of health , and we want to be able to use the technology safely. The acceptance of new technologies can be greatly impacted by the perceived security and privacy. Therefore, IMD designers should develop models of security and frameworks for thinking about the vulnerabilities that arise in their systems.

Security engineers should understand the key aspects of IMDs with special care on how data are issued and used and, hence, when/where/how vulnerabilities arise. Biosensors, and more generally IMDs, are complex systems that include information, physical, and human aspects. However, their small data rates and apparently simple functionality belie their emergent complexity that arises when considering the interface with the human body. We refrain from using the term *cyber-physical* due to its recent use emphasizing large-scale electromechanical systems such as power grids and transportation systems. Instead, we propose the term *cyber-human* to emphasize the role of humans in both the production and consumption of data. In both cases, the adversary is assumed to be human as well, and hence psychological, sociological, and even anthropological viewpoints need to be considered.

As computer security acquires more prominence in modern society, we expect that responsible citizens will need to invest time and effort in learning about vulnerabilities and defenses in IMDs, just as we do with more conventional crime, financial fraud, food safety, transportation security (from cars to airports), and personal safety. In all of these cases, new technologies have opened up opportunities for improved quality of life, but they have also opened up new vulnerabilities, especially for sophisticated attackers. One of the roles of local, national, and global governments should be to establish and enforce laws that allow for the best quality of life while minimizing the vulnerabilities. In many cases, market incentives can be used to help improve security, especially to augment those areas of life where government intervention is ineffective. Another self-regulating technique is the timely disclosure of security and data breach incidents and vulnerabilities. Researchers need to be allowed and incentivized to perform this important work without fear of unfair reprisal from device manufacturers or other legal hurdles.

Of course, all of this new demand proposes new challenges. Advances in biosensors and biodevices occur regularly. Reports of new scientific and technological advances related to medical devices appear continuously in the literature. New devices are announced regularly, and their acceptance by patients, physicians, insurers, and regulatory bodies continues to increase. New systems are regularly introduced to the market. New applications of sensors and devices emerge almost daily, even those that had not been considered previously when the devices were first produced. Unfortunately, the same can be said of the motivations, means, and effectiveness of malicious attacks.

New threats emerge continuously due to the increase in the accessibility of medical data previously unavailable or available only in specialized hospitals and labs (e.g., the information regarding patient genomics). Therefore, new defenses are now required, ranging from basic encryption and authentication to noncryptographic techniques such as jamming, shields, and firewalls. Any new protections need to address the related issues of costs, power budget limitations due to the portability of new devices, and the usability and reusability of the devices. From a still broader perspective, IMDs play a key role in higher-level health information systems. As a primary source of personal health data, IMDs will play a crucial role in defining new protocols for data gathering and new possibilities for malicious attacks and, thus, new actions for data protection. IMDs also provide a unique opportunity to tag data with a signature corresponding to its owner, date, time, location, and other information related to its origin.

To implement this vision, new policies, laws, ethics, and other aspects need to be jointly developed with the involvement of many sectors of modern society. Clearly, physicians, insurance companies, patients, governments, and other stakeholders need to be involved and to understand the tradeoffs between utility, safety, and costs. For example, if health insurance and, in turn, health care are mandated, how will this impact the rights of individuals to their health data? Several other related questions immediately arise. Which biological data are sensitive enough to require special protection? What information can be released to the public domain? What is fair for use? Who owns what data? and on and on. Therefore, technologists, physicians, lawyers, patients, government representatives, and other stakeholders need to be involved in this process of security and privacy development related to the new IMDs technologies that are so rapidly emerging now.

With this book, we hope to have started the now urgent process of addressing security and privacy in the field of IMDs by first soliciting the concerned scientists and technologists and raising awareness that now is the time to start working on the security and privacy issues while developing the new and powerful features of future IMDs.

References

1. J.T.B. Peterson, T.R. Deer, A History of Neurostimulation – in T.R.Deer at al., "Comprehensive Treatment of Chronic Pain by medical, Interventional, and Integrative Approaches", American Academy of Pain Medicine, 2013, DOI 10.1007/978-1-4614-1560-2_56
2. Margaret A. Hamburg, Francis S. Collins, The Path to Personalized Medicine, N Engl J Med 363(2010) 301–304
3. Sandro Carrara, Sara Seyedeh Ghoreishizadeh, Jacopo Olivo, Irene Taurino, Camilla Baj-Rossi, Andrea Cavallini, Maaike Op de Beeck, Catherine Dehollain, Wayne Burleson, Francis Gabriel Moussy, Anthony Guiseppi-Elie, Giovanni De Micheli, *Fully Integrated Biochip Platforms for Advanced Healthcare*, Sensors 12(2012) 11013–11060

Index

W. Burleson and S. Carrara (eds.), *Security and Privacy for Implantable Medical Devices*,
DOI 10.1007/978-1-4614-1674-6, © Springer Science+Business Media New York 2014

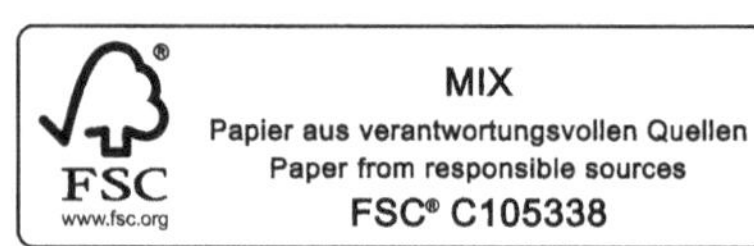

If you have any concerns about our products,
you can contact us on
ProductSafety@springernature.com

In case Publisher is established outside the EU,
the EU authorized representative is:
Springer Nature Customer Service Center GmbH
Europaplatz 3, 69115 Heidelberg, Germany

Printed by Libri Plureos GmbH
in Hamburg, Germany